Mometrix
TEST PREPARATION

Secrets of the

ARDMS®

Sonography Principles & Instrumentation Exam Study Guide

ARDMS and American Registry for Diagnostic Medical Sonography are registered trademarks of Intelios, Inc. The American Registry for Diagnostic Medical Sonography, Inc. (ARDMS) does not endorse this product nor is the ARDMS affiliated in any way with the owner or any content related to this product.

Disclaimer: The American Registry for Diagnostic Medical Sonography, Inc. (ARDMS) does not endorse this product nor is the ARDMS affiliated in any way with this product.

Dear Future Exam Success Story

First of all, **THANK YOU** for purchasing Mometrix study materials!

Second, congratulations! You are one of the few determined test-takers who are committed to doing whatever it takes to excel on your exam. **You have come to the right place.** We developed these study materials with one goal in mind: to deliver you the information you need in a format that's concise and easy to use.

In addition to optimizing your guide for the content of the test, we've outlined our recommended steps for breaking down the preparation process into small, attainable goals so you can make sure you stay on track.

We've also analyzed the entire test-taking process, identifying the most common pitfalls and showing how you can overcome them and be ready for any curveball the test throws you.

Standardized testing is one of the biggest obstacles on your road to success, which only increases the importance of doing well in the high-pressure, high-stakes environment of test day. Your results on this test could have a significant impact on your future, and this guide provides the information and practical advice to help you achieve your full potential on test day.

Your success is our success

We would love to hear from you! If you would like to share the story of your exam success or if you have any questions or comments in regard to our products, please contact us at **800-673-8175** or **support@mometrix.com**.

Thanks again for your business and we wish you continued success!

Sincerely,
The Mometrix Test Preparation Team

Need more help? Check out our flashcards at:
http://MometrixFlashcards.com/ARDMS

Copyright © 2026 by Mometrix Media LLC. All rights reserved.
Written and edited by the Mometrix Exam Secrets Test Prep Team
Printed in the United States of America

Table of Contents

- Introduction 1
- Secret Key 1: Plan Big, Study Small 2
- Secret Key 2: Make Your Studying Count 4
- Secret Key 3: Practice the Right Way 6
- Secret Key 4: Pace Yourself 8
- Secret Key 5: Have a Plan for Guessing 10
- Test-Taking Strategies 13
- Ultrasound Examinations 19
  - Patient Interactions 19
  - Patient Care and Safety 23
  - Interactions of Sound and Matter 27
  - Imaging Techniques 32
- Ultrasound Transducers 47
  - Transducer Components 47
  - Transducer Types 49
  - Transducer Selection 54
  - Transducer Assessment and Adjustment 55
- Optimizing Sonographic Images 58
  - Focus 58
  - Resolution 62
  - Magnification 67
  - Brightness 68
  - Depth 71
  - Duty Factor 72
  - Harmonic Imaging 73
  - M-Mode 74
  - Additional Imaging Techniques and Concepts 75
- Doppler Imaging 78
  - General Principles 78
  - Types of Doppler 84
  - Doppler Measurements 94
  - Artifacts 97
- Clinical Safety and Quality Assurance 99
  - Clinical Safety 99
  - Instrument Checks 101
  - Quality Assurance 104
- ARDMS Practice Test 107
- Answer Key and Explanations 128

IMAGE CREDITS	**153**
HOW TO OVERCOME TEST ANXIETY	**154**
ONLINE RESOURCES	**161**

Introduction

Thank you for purchasing this resource! You have made the choice to prepare yourself for a test that could have a huge impact on your future, and this guide is designed to help you be fully ready for test day. Obviously, it's important to have a solid understanding of the test material, but you also need to be prepared for the unique environment and stressors of the test, so that you can perform to the best of your abilities.

For this purpose, the first section that appears in this guide is the **Secret Keys**. We've devoted countless hours to meticulously researching what works and what doesn't, and we've boiled down our findings to the five most impactful steps you can take to improve your performance on the test. We start at the beginning with study planning and move through the preparation process, all the way to the testing strategies that will help you get the most out of what you know when you're finally sitting in front of the test.

We recommend that you start preparing for your test as far in advance as possible. However, if you've bought this guide as a last-minute study resource and only have a few days before your test, we recommend that you skip over the first two Secret Keys since they address a long-term study plan.

If you struggle with **test anxiety**, we strongly encourage you to check out our recommendations for how you can overcome it. Test anxiety is a formidable foe, but it can be beaten, and we want to make sure you have the tools you need to defeat it.

Secret Key 1: Plan Big, Study Small

There's a lot riding on your performance. If you want to ace this test, you're going to need to keep your skills sharp and the material fresh in your mind. You need a plan that lets you review everything you need to know while still fitting in your schedule. We'll break this strategy down into three categories.

Information Organization

Start with the information you already have: the official test outline. From this, you can make a complete list of all the concepts you need to cover before the test. Organize these concepts into groups that can be studied together, and create a list of any related vocabulary you need to learn so you can brush up on any difficult terms. You'll want to keep this vocabulary list handy once you actually start studying since you may need to add to it along the way.

Time Management

Once you have your set of study concepts, decide how to spread them out over the time you have left before the test. Break your study plan into small, clear goals so you have a manageable task for each day and know exactly what you're doing. Then just focus on one small step at a time. When you manage your time this way, you don't need to spend hours at a time studying. Studying a small block of content for a short period each day helps you retain information better and avoid stressing over how much you have left to do. You can relax knowing that you have a plan to cover everything in time. In order for this strategy to be effective though, you have to start studying early and stick to your schedule. Avoid the exhaustion and futility that comes from last-minute cramming!

Study Environment

The environment you study in has a big impact on your learning. Studying in a coffee shop, while probably more enjoyable, is not likely to be as fruitful as studying in a quiet room. It's important to keep distractions to a minimum. You're only planning to study for a short block of time, so make the most of it. Don't pause to check your phone or get up to find a snack. It's also important to **avoid multitasking**. Research has consistently shown that multitasking will make your studying dramatically less effective. Your study area should also be comfortable and well-lit so you don't have the distraction of straining your eyes or sitting on an uncomfortable chair.

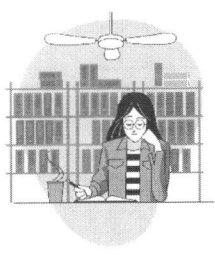 The time of day you study is also important. You want to be rested and alert. Don't wait until just before bedtime. Study when you'll be most likely to comprehend and remember. Even better, if you know what time of day your test will be, set that time aside for study. That way your brain will be used to working on that subject at that specific time and you'll have a better chance of recalling information.

Finally, it can be helpful to team up with others who are studying for the same test. Your actual studying should be done in as isolated an environment as possible, but the work of organizing the information and setting up the study plan can be divided up. In between study sessions, you can discuss with your teammates the concepts that you're all studying and quiz each other on the details. Just be sure that your teammates are as serious about the test as you are. If you find that your study time is being replaced with social time, you might need to find a new team.

Secret Key 2: Make Your Studying Count

You're devoting a lot of time and effort to preparing for this test, so you want to be absolutely certain it will pay off. This means doing more than just reading the content and hoping you can remember it on test day. It's important to make every minute of study count. There are two main areas you can focus on to make your studying count.

Retention

It doesn't matter how much time you study if you can't remember the material. You need to make sure you are retaining the concepts. To check your retention of the information you're learning, try recalling it at later times with minimal prompting. Try carrying around flashcards and glance at one or two from time to time or ask a friend who's also studying for the test to quiz you.

To enhance your retention, look for ways to put the information into practice so that you can apply it rather than simply recalling it. If you're using the information in practical ways, it will be much easier to remember. Similarly, it helps to solidify a concept in your mind if you're not only reading it to yourself but also explaining it to someone else. Ask a friend to let you teach them about a concept you're a little shaky on (or speak aloud to an imaginary audience if necessary). As you try to summarize, define, give examples, and answer your friend's questions, you'll understand the concepts better and they will stay with you longer. Finally, step back for a big picture view and ask yourself how each piece of information fits with the whole subject. When you link the different concepts together and see them working together as a whole, it's easier to remember the individual components.

Finally, practice showing your work on any multi-step problems, even if you're just studying. Writing out each step you take to solve a problem will help solidify the process in your mind, and you'll be more likely to remember it during the test.

Modality

Modality simply refers to the means or method by which you study. Choosing a study modality that fits your own individual learning style is crucial. No two people learn best in exactly the same way, so it's important to know your strengths and use them to your advantage.

For example, if you learn best by visualization, focus on visualizing a concept in your mind and draw an image or a diagram. Try color-coding your notes, illustrating them, or creating symbols that will trigger your mind to recall a learned concept. If you learn best by hearing or discussing information, find a study partner who learns the same way or read aloud to yourself. Think about how to put the information in your own words. Imagine that you are giving a lecture on the topic and record yourself so you can listen to it later.

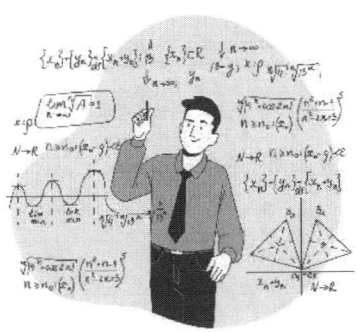

For any learning style, flashcards can be helpful. Organize the information so you can take advantage of spare moments to review. Underline key words or phrases. Use different colors for different categories. Mnemonic devices (such as creating a short list in which every item starts with the same letter) can also help with retention. Find what works best for you and use it to store the information in your mind most effectively and easily.

Secret Key 3: Practice the Right Way

Your success on test day depends not only on how many hours you put into preparing, but also on whether you prepared the right way. It's good to check along the way to see if your studying is paying off. One of the most effective ways to do this is by taking practice tests to evaluate your progress. Practice tests are useful because they show exactly where you need to improve. Every time you take a practice test, pay special attention to these three groups of questions:

- The questions you got wrong
- The questions you had to guess on, even if you guessed right
- The questions you found difficult or slow to work through

This will show you exactly what your weak areas are, and where you need to devote more study time. Ask yourself why each of these questions gave you trouble. Was it because you didn't understand the material? Was it because you didn't remember the vocabulary? Do you need more repetitions on this type of question to build speed and confidence? Dig into those questions and figure out how you can strengthen your weak areas as you go back to review the material.

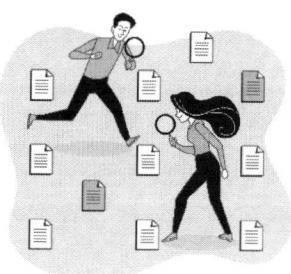

Additionally, many practice tests have a section explaining the answer choices. It can be tempting to read the explanation and think that you now have a good understanding of the concept. However, an explanation likely only covers part of the question's broader context. Even if the explanation makes perfect sense, **go back and investigate** every concept related to the question until you're positive you have a thorough understanding.

As you go along, keep in mind that the practice test is just that: practice. Memorizing these questions and answers will not be very helpful on the actual test because it is unlikely to have any of the same exact questions. If you only know the right answers to the sample questions, you won't be prepared for the real thing. **Study the concepts** until you understand them fully, and then you'll be able to answer any question that shows up on the test.

It's important to wait on the practice tests until you're ready. If you take a test on your first day of study, you may be overwhelmed by the amount of material covered and how much you need to learn. Work up to it gradually.

On test day, you'll need to be prepared for answering questions, managing your time, and using the test-taking strategies you've learned. It's a lot to balance, like a mental marathon that will have a big impact on your future. Like training for a marathon, you'll need to start slowly and work your way up. When test day arrives, you'll be ready.

Start with the strategies you've read in the first two Secret Keys—plan your course and study in the way that works best for you. If you have time, consider using multiple study resources to get different approaches to the same concepts. It can be helpful to see difficult concepts from more than one angle. Then find a good source for practice tests. Many times, the test website will suggest potential study resources or provide sample tests.

Practice Test Strategy

If you're able to find at least three practice tests, we recommend this strategy:

UNTIMED AND OPEN-BOOK PRACTICE

Take the first test with no time constraints and with your notes and study guide handy. Take your time and focus on applying the strategies you've learned.

TIMED AND OPEN-BOOK PRACTICE

Take the second practice test open-book as well, but set a timer and practice pacing yourself to finish in time.

TIMED AND CLOSED-BOOK PRACTICE

Take any other practice tests as if it were test day. Set a timer and put away your study materials. Sit at a table or desk in a quiet room, imagine yourself at the testing center, and answer questions as quickly and accurately as possible.

Keep repeating timed and closed-book tests on a regular basis until you run out of practice tests or it's time for the actual test. Your mind will be ready for the schedule and stress of test day, and you'll be able to focus on recalling the material you've learned.

Secret Key 4: Pace Yourself

Once you're fully prepared for the material on the test, your biggest challenge on test day will be managing your time. Just knowing that the clock is ticking can make you panic even if you have plenty of time left. Work on pacing yourself so you can build confidence against the time constraints of the exam. Pacing is a difficult skill to master, especially in a high-pressure environment, so **practice is vital**.

Set time expectations for your pace based on how much time is available. For example, if a section has 60 questions and the time limit is 30 minutes, you know you have to average 30 seconds or less per question in order to answer them all. Although 30 seconds is the hard limit, set 25 seconds per question as your goal, so you reserve extra time to spend on harder questions. When you budget extra time for the harder questions, you no longer have any reason to stress when those questions take longer to answer.

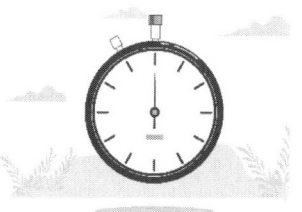

Don't let this time expectation distract you from working through the test at a calm, steady pace, but keep it in mind so you don't spend too much time on any one question. Recognize that taking extra time on one question you don't understand may keep you from answering two that you do understand later in the test. If your time limit for a question is up and you're still not sure of the answer, mark it and move on, and come back to it later if the time and the test format allow. If the testing format doesn't allow you to return to earlier questions, just make an educated guess; then put it out of your mind and move on.

On the easier questions, be careful not to rush. It may seem wise to hurry through them so you have more time for the challenging ones, but it's not worth missing one if you know the concept and just didn't take the time to read the question fully. Work efficiently but make sure you understand the question and have looked at all of the answer choices, since more than one may seem right at first.

Even if you're paying attention to the time, you may find yourself a little behind at some point. You should speed up to get back on track, but do so wisely. Don't panic; just take a few seconds less on each question until you're caught up. Don't guess without thinking, but do look through the answer choices and eliminate any you know are wrong. If you can get down to two choices, it is often worthwhile to guess from those. Once you've chosen an answer, move on and don't dwell on any that you skipped or had to hurry through. If a question was taking too long, chances are it was one of the harder ones, so you weren't as likely to get it right anyway.

On the other hand, if you find yourself getting ahead of schedule, it may be beneficial to slow down a little. The more quickly you work, the more likely you are to make a careless mistake that will affect your score. You've budgeted time for each question, so don't be afraid to spend that time. Practice an efficient but careful pace to get the most out of the time you have.

Secret Key 5: Have a Plan for Guessing

When you're taking the test, you may find yourself stuck on a question. Some of the answer choices seem better than others, but you don't see the one answer choice that is obviously correct. What do you do?

The scenario described above is very common, yet most test takers have not effectively prepared for it. Developing and practicing a plan for guessing may be one of the single most effective uses of your time as you get ready for the exam.

In developing your plan for guessing, there are three questions to address:

- When should you start the guessing process?
- How should you narrow down the choices?
- Which answer should you choose?

When to Start the Guessing Process

Unless your plan for guessing is to select C every time (which, despite its merits, is not what we recommend), you need to leave yourself enough time to apply your answer elimination strategies. Since you have a limited amount of time for each question, that means that if you're going to give yourself the best shot at guessing correctly, you have to decide quickly whether or not you will guess.

Of course, the best-case scenario is that you don't have to guess at all, so first, see if you can answer the question based on your knowledge of the subject and basic reasoning skills. Focus on the key words in the question and try to jog your memory of related topics. Give yourself a chance to bring the knowledge to mind, but once you realize that you don't have (or you can't access) the knowledge you need to answer the question, it's time to start the guessing process.

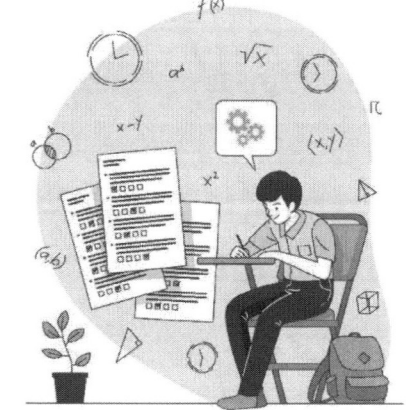

It's almost always better to start the guessing process too early than too late. It only takes a few seconds to remember something and answer the question from knowledge. Carefully eliminating wrong answer choices takes longer. Plus, going through the process of eliminating answer choices can actually help jog your memory.

Summary: Start the guessing process as soon as you decide that you can't answer the question based on your knowledge.

How to Narrow Down the Choices

The next chapter in this book (**Test-Taking Strategies**) includes a wide range of strategies for how to approach questions and how to look for answer choices to eliminate. You will definitely want to read those carefully, practice them, and figure out which ones work best for you. Here though, we're going to address a mindset rather than a particular strategy.

Your odds of guessing an answer correctly depend on how many options you are choosing from.

Number of options left	5	4	3	2	1
Odds of guessing correctly	20%	25%	33%	50%	100%

You can see from this chart just how valuable it is to be able to eliminate incorrect answers and make an educated guess, but there are two things that many test takers do that cause them to miss out on the benefits of guessing:

- Accidentally eliminating the correct answer
- Selecting an answer based on an impression

We'll look at the first one here, and the second one in the next section.

To avoid accidentally eliminating the correct answer, we recommend a thought exercise called **the $5 challenge**. In this challenge, you only eliminate an answer choice from contention if you are willing to bet $5 on it being wrong. Why $5? Five dollars is a small but not insignificant amount of money. It's an amount you could afford to lose but wouldn't want to throw away. And while losing $5 once might not hurt too much, doing it twenty times will set you back $100. In the same way, each small decision you make—eliminating a choice here, guessing on a question there—won't by itself impact your score very much, but when you put them all together, they can make a big difference. By holding each answer choice elimination decision to a higher standard, you can reduce the risk of accidentally eliminating the correct answer.

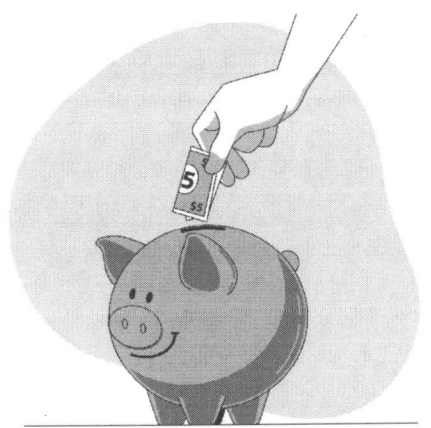

The $5 challenge can also be applied in a positive sense: If you are willing to bet $5 that an answer choice *is* correct, go ahead and mark it as correct.

Summary: Only eliminate an answer choice if you are willing to bet $5 that it is wrong.

Which Answer to Choose

You're taking the test. You've run into a hard question and decided you'll have to guess. You've eliminated all the answer choices you're willing to bet $5 on. Now you have to pick an answer. Why do we even need to talk about this? Why can't you just pick whichever one you feel like when the time comes?

The answer to these questions is that if you don't come into the test with a plan, you'll rely on your impression to select an answer choice, and if you do that, you risk falling into a trap. The test writers know that everyone who takes their test will be guessing on some of the questions, so they intentionally write wrong answer choices to seem plausible. You still have to pick an answer though, and if the wrong answer choices are designed to look right, how can you ever be sure that you're not falling for their trap? The best solution we've found to this dilemma is to take the decision out of your hands entirely. Here is the process we recommend:

Once you've eliminated any choices that you are confident (willing to bet $5) are wrong, select the first remaining choice as your answer.

Whether you choose to select the first remaining choice, the second, or the last, the important thing is that you use some preselected standard. Using this approach guarantees that you will not be enticed into selecting an answer choice that looks right, because you are not basing your decision on how the answer choices look.

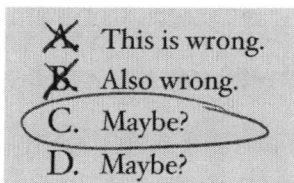

This is not meant to make you question your knowledge. Instead, it is to help you recognize the difference between your knowledge and your impressions. There's a huge difference between thinking an answer is right because of what you know, and thinking an answer is right because it looks or sounds like it should be right.

Summary: To ensure that your selection is appropriately random, make a predetermined selection from among all answer choices you have not eliminated.

Test-Taking Strategies

This section contains a list of test-taking strategies that you may find helpful as you work through the test. By taking what you know and applying logical thought, you can maximize your chances of answering any question correctly!

It is very important to realize that every question is different and every person is different: no single strategy will work on every question, and no single strategy will work for every person. That's why we've included all of them here, so you can try them out and determine which ones work best for different types of questions and which ones work best for you.

Question Strategies

✓ Read Carefully

Read the question and the answer choices carefully. Don't miss the question because you misread the terms. You have plenty of time to read each question thoroughly and make sure you understand what is being asked. Yet a happy medium must be attained, so don't waste too much time. You must read carefully and efficiently.

✓ Contextual Clues

Look for contextual clues. If the question includes a word you are not familiar with, look at the immediate context for some indication of what the word might mean. Contextual clues can often give you all the information you need to decipher the meaning of an unfamiliar word. Even if you can't determine the meaning, you may be able to narrow down the possibilities enough to make a solid guess at the answer to the question.

✓ Prefixes

If you're having trouble with a word in the question or answer choices, try dissecting it. Take advantage of every clue that the word might include. Prefixes can be a huge help. Usually, they allow you to determine a basic meaning. *Pre-* means before, *post-* means after, *pro-* is positive, *de-* is negative. From prefixes, you can get an idea of the general meaning of the word and try to put it into context.

✓ Hedge Words

Watch out for critical hedge words, such as *likely, may, can, often, almost, mostly, usually, generally, rarely,* and *sometimes*. Question writers insert these hedge phrases to cover every possibility. Often an answer choice will be wrong simply because it leaves no room for exception. Be on guard for answer choices that have definitive words such as *exactly* and *always*.

⊘ Switchback Words

Stay alert for *switchbacks*. These are the words and phrases frequently used to alert you to shifts in thought. The most common switchback words are *but, although*, and *however*. Others include *nevertheless, on the other hand, even though, while, in spite of, despite*, and *regardless of*. Switchback words are important to catch because they can change the direction of the question or an answer choice.

⊘ Face Value

When in doubt, use common sense. Accept the situation in the problem at face value. Don't read too much into it. These problems will not require you to make wild assumptions. If you have to go beyond creativity and warp time or space in order to have an answer choice fit the question, then you should move on and consider the other answer choices. These are normal problems rooted in reality. The applicable relationship or explanation may not be readily apparent, but it is there for you to figure out. Use your common sense to interpret anything that isn't clear.

Answer Choice Strategies

⊘ Answer Selection

The most thorough way to pick an answer choice is to identify and eliminate wrong answers until only one is left, then confirm it is the correct answer. Sometimes an answer choice may immediately seem right, but be careful. The test writers will usually put more than one reasonable answer choice on each question, so take a second to read all of them and make sure that the other choices are not equally obvious. As long as you have time left, it is better to read every answer choice than to pick the first one that looks right without checking the others.

⊘ Answer Choice Families

An answer choice family consists of two (in rare cases, three) answer choices that are very similar in construction and cannot all be true at the same time. If you see two answer choices that are direct opposites or parallels, one of them is usually the correct answer. For instance, if one answer choice says that quantity x increases and another either says that quantity x decreases (opposite) or says that quantity y increases (parallel), then those answer choices would fall into the same family. An answer choice that doesn't match the construction of the answer choice family is more likely to be incorrect. Most questions will not have answer choice families, but when they do appear, you should be prepared to recognize them.

⊘ Eliminate Answers

Eliminate answer choices as soon as you realize they are wrong, but make sure you consider all possibilities. If you are eliminating answer choices and realize that the last one you are left with is also wrong, don't panic. Start over and consider each choice again. There may be something you missed the first time that you will realize on the second pass.

⊘ Avoid Fact Traps

Don't be distracted by an answer choice that is factually true but doesn't answer the question. You are looking for the choice that answers the question. Stay focused on what the question is asking for so you don't accidentally pick an answer that is true but incorrect. Always go back to the question and make sure the answer choice you've selected actually answers the question and is not merely a true statement.

⊘ Extreme Statements

In general, you should avoid answers that put forth extreme actions as standard practice or proclaim controversial ideas as established fact. An answer choice that states the "process should be used in certain situations, if..." is much more likely to be correct than one that states the "process should be discontinued completely." The first is a calm rational statement and doesn't even make a definitive, uncompromising stance, using a hedge word *if* to provide wiggle room, whereas the second choice is far more extreme.

⊘ Benchmark

As you read through the answer choices and you come across one that seems to answer the question well, mentally select that answer choice. This is not your final answer, but it's the one that will help you evaluate the other answer choices. The one that you selected is your benchmark or standard for judging each of the other answer choices. Every other answer choice must be compared to your benchmark. That choice is correct until proven otherwise by another answer choice beating it. If you find a better answer, then that one becomes your new benchmark. Once you've decided that no other choice answers the question as well as your benchmark, you have your final answer.

⊘ Predict the Answer

Before you even start looking at the answer choices, it is often best to try to predict the answer. When you come up with the answer on your own, it is easier to avoid distractions and traps because you will know exactly what to look for. The right answer choice is unlikely to be word-for-word what you came up with, but it should be a close match. Even if you are confident that you have the right answer, you should still take the time to read each option before moving on.

General Strategies

⊘ Tough Questions

If you are stumped on a problem or it appears too hard or too difficult, don't waste time. Move on! Remember though, if you can quickly check for obviously incorrect answer choices, your chances of guessing correctly are greatly improved. Before you completely give up, at least try to knock out a couple of possible answers. Eliminate what you can and then guess at the remaining answer choices before moving on.

✓ Check Your Work

Since you will probably not know every term listed and the answer to every question, it is important that you get credit for the ones that you do know. Don't miss any questions through careless mistakes. If at all possible, try to take a second to look back over your answer selection and make sure you've selected the correct answer choice and haven't made a costly careless mistake (such as marking an answer choice that you didn't mean to mark). This quick double check should more than pay for itself in caught mistakes for the time it costs.

✓ Pace Yourself

It's easy to be overwhelmed when you're looking at a page full of questions; your mind is confused and full of random thoughts, and the clock is ticking down faster than you would like. Calm down and maintain the pace that you have set for yourself. Especially as you get down to the last few minutes of the test, don't let the small numbers on the clock make you panic. As long as you are on track by monitoring your pace, you are guaranteed to have time for each question.

✓ Don't Rush

It is very easy to make errors when you are in a hurry. Maintaining a fast pace in answering questions is pointless if it makes you miss questions that you would have gotten right otherwise. Test writers like to include distracting information and wrong answers that seem right. Taking a little extra time to avoid careless mistakes can make all the difference in your test score. Find a pace that allows you to be confident in the answers that you select.

✓ Keep Moving

Panicking will not help you pass the test, so do your best to stay calm and keep moving. Taking deep breaths and going through the answer elimination steps you practiced can help to break through a stress barrier and keep your pace.

Final Notes

The combination of a solid foundation of content knowledge and the confidence that comes from practicing your plan for applying that knowledge is the key to maximizing your performance on test day. As your foundation of content knowledge is built up and strengthened, you'll find that the strategies included in this chapter become more and more effective in helping you quickly sift through the distractions and traps of the test to isolate the correct answer.

Now that you're preparing to move forward into the test content chapters of this book, be sure to keep your goal in mind. As you read, think about how you will be able to apply this information on the test. If you've already seen sample questions for the test and you have an idea of the question format and style, try to come up with questions of your own that you can answer based on what you're reading. This will give you valuable practice applying your knowledge in the same ways you can expect to on test day.

Good luck and good studying!

Ultrasound Examinations

Patient Interactions

INFORMED CONSENT

In any clinical role, it is important to obtain a patient's informed consent. **Informed consent** is the process of providing clear and comprehensive information about a medical procedure, treatment, or intervention and an explanation of why it is necessary. It allows them to use this information to make an educated, voluntary decision about whether they want to proceed with the suggested course of action. The patient's level of comprehension should be assessed so that this information can be presented in an appropriate manner. It is important to consider any cultural or language barriers that may be in place. Cultural differences require a high degree of sensitivity because a patient's culture can have a large impact on medical comprehension and decision making. If significant language barriers are encountered, the use of an interpreter or translator may be necessary. Patients have the right to decline the medical procedure as well as withdraw their previously provided consent.

As a sonographer, informed consent emphasizes the importance of communication, respect for patient autonomy, and patient-centered care. In addition to explaining the ultrasound procedure, it is critical to reinforce the fact that ultrasound is considered a safe, noninvasive means of imaging and does not involve ionizing radiation. If the patient refuses the exam or withdraws previously provided consent at any time, the sonographer must respect and acknowledge this decision without judgment or pressure. This decision should also be communicated to the healthcare team and should be appropriately documented.

INITIAL PATIENT ENCOUNTER

An ultrasound exam encounter should always begin with a warm greeting, along with an **introduction** of the ultrasound technologist and their role in the exam. Then, the **patient's identity** should always be confirmed using unique identifiers such as their full name along with date of birth. This can be done verbally or by checking a medical wristband, if present. All details provided should be cross checked with the details in their medical records or ultrasound system.

Once patient identity is verified, the purpose of the ordered exam should be clearly explained, avoiding medical jargon as much as possible. It is important to ensure that the patient completely understands the procedure as well as any risks or benefits. Any concerns should be promptly addressed to ensure optimal comfort and to **build rapport**.

The **patient's medical history** should always be reviewed prior to the exam to check for any preexisting conditions or relevant history. Questions should be asked relating to the examination to ensure accuracy and safety. For example, if a patient with a contrast allergy requires a vascular ultrasound, then the sonographer can review the medical history and be sure to avoid contrast administration and reduce the chance of complications.

In conjunction with the patient's history, it is equally important to assess the **appropriateness of the ordered imaging study** and its alignment with the patient's symptoms and condition. This enables the sonographer to justify that the exam is necessary and meaningfully contributes to a patient's diagnosis and treatment. Avoiding unnecessary imaging studies ensures cost-effectiveness and that healthcare resources are being efficiently used. Additionally, it minimizes a patient's unnecessary exposure to ultrasound, coinciding with the ALARA principle.

Clinical History and Previous Imaging Studies

Often, an ultrasound exam may be performed as a follow-up to a disorder that has already been diagnosed with another imaging modality or a prior ultrasound study. If a patient has had prior imaging (e.g., magnetic resonance imaging [MRI], computed tomography [CT], ultrasound, etc.), it is important to look at the images and read the report so that the sonographer knows exactly what is to be interrogated. It is also important that the radiologist has this information because ordering physicians appreciate and expect comparative reports. Ultrasound is useful as a follow-up modality because it does not subject the patient to ionizing radiation like CT and x-ray do. The facility may use a technique called fusion imaging, which allows side-by-side ultrasound imaging with comparative CT or MRI studies that have already been performed. This technique allows for greater confidence that the lesion visualized on ultrasound is the exact same lesion found on a previous study.

Review Medical and Surgical History

Reviewing a patient's medical or surgical history is an important process to gather relevant data before beginning any medical exam. A patient's history can include crucial details about potential risks that may have an impact on the procedure. Sonographers need to be aware of these risks or complications so that the ultrasound exam or imaging protocol can be adapted to the patient's needs.

Implants or other medical devices can affect the clarity of an ultrasound image. Being aware of this can aid the sonographer in understanding why certain structures may not be easily visualized. Having knowledge of previous surgeries or medical conditions is therefore crucial. This allows for sonographers to tailor the imaging protocol based on the patient's condition. Imagine needing to perform an abdominal ultrasound of the right upper quadrant and realizing that the patient had a surgical history of cholecystectomy (i.e., gallbladder removal). The sonographer would then not need to waste time on obtaining images of the gallbladder.

Although reviewing the history is important for the exam itself, it also has an empathetic component. A patient who feels heard and understood is more likely to have a positive healthcare experience. Inquiring about the patient's prior history builds trust and contributes to a holistic approach to patient care. It shows that the sonographer is fully committed to understanding the individual's overall health.

Understanding and reviewing a patient's past medical history is pivotal in healthcare, ensuring diagnostic accuracy, safety, and patient-centered care.

Patient Communication During an Ultrasound Exam

It is important to show empathy during an ultrasound exam. Often, the patient is nervous about the procedure, so it is up to the sonographer to help the patient feel more comfortable. Upon having correctly identified the patient, the sonographer should introduce themself to the patient, explain the exam that will be performed, and answer any questions that may arise. An important step prior to the exam is to get a thorough history from the patient and find out if any prior exams have been done for comparison. Make sure that the patient is as comfortable as possible, and during the exam check in and ask him/her how they are doing. Once the exam is complete, make sure that all of the gel is wiped off. It is also important to discuss how the patient will receive their results and when to expect them. A sonographer should not relay any of the associated findings with the patient because results must come from the ordering physician or radiologist. Patients often appreciate being shown back to the waiting room after the exam is finished.

Confidentiality and Privacy Guidelines

Confidentiality and privacy are crucial to the ethical practice of ultrasound. Patients undergoing ultrasound examinations have the right to privacy, confidentiality, and autonomy. This is essential for building patient trust and upholding the integrity of the sonography profession.

Various ultrasound examinations will require an extra privacy measure. For example, some OB ultrasounds involve transvaginal probes, which require insertion into the vaginal canal. This is where respecting patient privacy is critical. The use of appropriate drapes as well as establishing clear communication with the patient about the procedure will contribute to patient comfort. Privacy screens or curtains in examination rooms should also be used as a physical barrier. This will further enhance a feeling of privacy.

It is also important to ensure a private discussion space before and after an exam. Patients will often have questions or concerns, and they are better able to express themselves in a confidential and private setting. It is the responsibility of the sonographer to implement privacy measures to foster a safe space.

Securing patient data is also a key component of maintaining confidentiality and privacy in the healthcare setting. Patients' medical records, ultrasound images, and other medical data should be stored and transmitted in a secure fashion.

Sonographers must ensure that a patient's medical information always remains private. Safeguarding ultrasound images and sensitive details is paramount, and this information should only be accessible by authorized healthcare professionals.

HIPAA

The Health Insurance Portability and Accountability Act of 1996 (HIPAA) is the framework of patient confidentiality and privacy. Sonographers should always prioritize adherence to HIPAA regulations, ensuring that the electronic and physical storage of ultrasound data and private health information is secure.

GENERAL PATIENT CARE STANDARDS

General patient care should include the following elements:

- **Clear communication**—During patient interactions, it is critical to maintain a professional demeanor and establish clear communication. Explain the ultrasound procedure in detail, addressing any concerns or questions that the patient may have. Clear communication with the ordering physician, as well as any healthcare professional associated with a patient's care, is also important.
- **Privacy and dignity**—Ultrasound examinations can be extremely sensitive; therefore, upholding the dignity of the patient is the sonographer's responsibility. The appropriate draping for various ultrasound exams should always be provided. Respect for patient privacy and dignity fosters trust and a positive healthcare experience.
- **Patient comfort**—When someone comes to the hospital or clinic, they are typically anxious. Ensuring a comfortable and safe ultrasound environment helps to decrease this anxiety. Special attention should also be given to patients expressing signs of discomfort or pain, making sure to use different techniques as needed to enhance patient comfort and cooperation.
- **Infection control**—Sonographers should adhere to infection control protocols such as proper hand hygiene, the donning of appropriate personal protective equipment (PPE), and disinfection of medical equipment. This will minimize the risk of infections being spread among healthcare workers as well as patients.

Patient Care and Safety

ALARA Principle

The as low as reasonably achievable (ALARA) principle is associated with radiation, but it is also an important rule for sonographers. It is the concept of minimizing a patient's exposure to ultrasound energy while maintaining diagnostic quality. For example, if an entire image is too bright, the most effective way to decrease patient exposure is to decrease the output power (also known as the acoustic power). By lowering the power, there is a decrease in the voltage applied to the ultrasound transducer, which, in turn, decreases the amount of energy that the patient is exposed to. A sonographer could also turn down the overall gain to prevent an image from being too bright but should understand that gain has no effect on patient exposure. However, if an image is too dark, the best choice for adhering to the ALARA principle is to increase the gain because it does not affect the energy imparted to the patient.

Impact of Highly Focused Beam

A highly focused ultrasound beam can produce a greater degree of internal tissue heating because the energy of the beam is condensed into a thin region, especially at the focus where the beam diameter is already the smallest. Although this has a positive effect on image resolution, it may increase the temperature of the internal tissue. Tissue heating relates to the spatial peak temporal average (SPTA) intensity. This is a value that should be watched closely by the operator, especially during fetal scans because bioeffects must be taken into consideration. When compared to an unfocused beam, a focused beam is allowed to have a higher SPTA intensity limit because less tissue is being exposed. The intensity limit of a focused beam is set at 1 W/cm^2 or 1,000 mW/cm^2.

Elevation in Temperature of Tissues

Ultrasound should only be used for clinical exams in which the benefits outweigh the risks. One risk during an exam is an elevation of temperature in tissues exposed to the ultrasound beam. The thermal index (TI) will be highest during an exam with a high-frequency, high-intensity beam. This heating depends on exposure time and temperature. Typically, the greatest increase in temperature is witnessed with spectral Doppler exams. Pulsed-wave Doppler requires more energy than B-mode or grayscale imaging. Ideally, the TI should be 1.0 or less and the time should be minimized to prevent tissue heating. If the TI is 1.0, this means that there is a possibility that the temperature of the tissues will increase by 1 °C. TI is expressed by the soft-tissue thermal index, bone thermal index, and cranial bone thermal index.

Intensity Limits for Unfocused and Focused Ultrasound

During an exam, the sonographer must keep the range of output intensity (or the energy of the ultrasound beam) within an acceptable level to reduce the chances of bioeffects. During an ultrasound study, the sonographer must be aware of the output intensity (or energy) of the ultrasound beam in order to reduce the risk of bioeffects to the patient. This intensity is called the spatial peak temporal average (SPTA), and it is the most pertinent intensity with regard to tissue heating. If an unfocused ultrasound beam is used, there must be a lower intensity limit set versus if a focused transducer is used. An unfocused beam is wider, and it allows more ultrasound energy to reach a greater cross-sectional area of tissue. Therefore, to compensate for the wide beam exposure to the patient, 100 mW/cm^2 is used for the intensity threshold of an unfocused beam. A focused beam intensity limit, which exposes less tissue to the energy of the ultrasound beam, is safely set at 1 W/cm^2 or 1,000 mW/cm^2.

ERGONOMIC TECHNIQUES

PROPER ERGONOMICS IN ULTRASOUND LABS

Ultrasound managers are aware of the astronomical costs associated with new employee hiring, training, and worker's compensation claims. Ergonomics awareness is a must in the ultrasound lab in order to maintain a sonographer's health and avoid work-related musculoskeletal injuries. Often, these injuries are career ending (20%), and almost 75% of sonographers tend to have symptoms of pain, numbness, tingling, and swelling to some degree. These symptoms do not occur only while scanning; they may also be felt throughout the day and while away from the lab. These injuries are difficult to treat especially if sonographers continue to scan in the same way. Employers must make sure that their staff has the equipment necessary to prevent these injuries from occurring along with continuing education concerning these risk factors. An imaging manager should allow for breaks between ultrasound exams to give each employee time to stretch. The number of exams performed by each sonographer should be limited so that injuries do not occur as a result of inadequate rest time. The ultrasound lab should be equipped with ergonomic tables and chairs, and the ultrasound machine itself should be adjusted so that staff can safely and comfortably perform exams.

KNOWLEDGE OF ERGONOMICS

To reduce the risk of work-related musculoskeletal disorders, sonographers should prioritize ergonomics because it is beneficial to their long-term health. Repetitive tasks that are performed during ultrasounds tend to contribute to physical strain and stresses among technologists. The sonography workspace and technical equipment should be arranged appropriately so that sonographers can navigate with ease and comfort.

The ultrasound machine's placement has a direct impact on the body, especially the back, neck, and shoulders. It should therefore be adjusted to an appropriate height and angle so that the sonographer does not spend a lot of time bending, reaching, or twisting. Adjusting the patient's bed, if possible, can also be helpful to avoid awkward positions and uncomfortable scanning.

Ultrasound departments should emphasize the importance of breaks as well as stretching exercises to help alleviate stress, strain, and tension. Ergonomic training programs or exercises can also be helpful to allow for continuing education and improvement. Adhering to ergonomic protocols and best practices enhances workplace productivity, job satisfaction, and overall well-being.

BIOEFFECTS

MAMMALIAN BIOEFFECTS OF ULTRASOUND IN VIVO

The term in vivo involves observing possible bioeffects that take place inside a living body. The spatial peak temporal average (SPTA) is the intensity referred to in the Statement on Mammalian Biological Effects of Ultrasound In Vivo of the American Institute of Ultrasound in Medicine. Unfavorable outcomes have been observed in exploratory conditions. Many experiments have been carried out in the lab setting pertaining to the possible bioeffects that ultrasound has on the body. Lab mammals are used to help experts better comprehend the associated risks that ultrasound has on the body. Lower ultrasound frequencies pose no threat to human tissue during in vivo trials. During controlled trials, it has been confirmed that as long as a focused beam's SPTA intensity does not exceed 1 W/cm^2 and an unfocused beam's SPTA intensity stays less than 100 mW/cm^2, then bioeffects should not occur.

EPIDEMIOLOGICAL STUDIES OF BIOEFFECTS

In order to determine the safety of ultrasound exams, many epidemiological studies have been performed. These studies evaluate if any associated bioeffects were found when the patient was exposed to ultrasound in utero. Thousands of women are scanned every year as part of a routine obstetric (OB) workup, and poor outcomes cannot be connected with the use of ultrasound during pregnancy. There are drawbacks to the epidemiological approach. For example, the fetal environment in is not considered. Low birth weight, delayed speech, and short stature may be caused by smoking and drug and alcohol abuse and not interrogation in utero with ultrasound. These studies do not look at how many times or how long the patient was exposed to ultrasound or why the exam was performed.

MECHANICAL INDEX

The mechanical index (MI) reading on an ultrasound machine determines the probability of bioeffects when gas bubbles in the tissue interact with the ultrasound beam. This is a phenomenon known as cavitation. The significance of a system displaying a high MI is that there is a better chance that bioeffects will occur. If a sonographer notices that the MI is too high, it is helpful to decrease the output power on the machine in order to reduce the amount of voltage sent to the transducer. The operator should also increase the frequency of the transducer because the frequency and MI have an inverse relationship. These adjustments are effective in reducing the display because lower frequency and pressure are two properties of the beam that tend to raise the MI.

CAVITATION

The two types of cavitation that exist when the force and frequency from an ultrasound beam are applied to tissues are known as stable cavitation and transient cavitation. The mechanical index (MI) reading on the machine alerts the sonographer to the possibility that cavitation will create dangerous bioeffects within the tissue being imaged. A smaller MI number indicates that stable cavitation will occur. Stable cavitation is the increasing, decreasing, and vibration of gas bubbles located within tissue when it is exposed to variations in pressure of the sound wave. These bubbles tend to acquire much of the energy of the sound wave, but they do not rupture. Transient (normal, inertial) cavitation occurs with higher MI readings. In this situation, the microbubbles tend to rupture, creating increased pressure and temperature.

Monitoring the Thermal Index

Patient safety is a primary concern during an ultrasound. Bioeffects can occur if an increase in tissue temperature occurs as a result of the interactions of tissue with the ultrasound beam. The thermal index (TI) is displayed on the screen for users as an indicator of a possible increase in tissue temperature. Research has shown that an increase in temperature of some tissues by as little as 2–4 °C can cause bioeffects. Of course, this heating depends on the tissue type as well as the amount of time the tissue is exposed. The TI is directly related to the acoustic output of the machine. There are three types of TIs that serve as the best in vivo indicators of a rise in temperature: the soft-tissue thermal index, bone thermal index, and cranial bone thermal index. Obstetric exams are of great concern because adverse effects have been identified with an elevated TI value.

Achieving the Lowest TI

It is no surprise that the lowest level of tissue heating occurs when the output intensity of the equipment being used is at its lowest numerical value. Generally, grayscale imaging is the method in which tissue heating will be the lowest. Tissue heating is typically the highest when pulsed Doppler is being used. M-mode and color flow Doppler tend to fall in the middle of these intensities. One way to determine the numerical values of these intensities is to evaluate the sound wave by using a hydrophone. A hydrophone may be used by engineers to measure the output intensities as well as other characteristics of an ultrasound wave. The hydrophone is actually a transducer that is about the size of a needle that provides accurate values because of its compact size.

Obtaining the Fetal Heart Rate During the First Trimester

The best method of obtaining the fetal heart rate with ultrasound during the first trimester is with M-mode (also referred to as motion mode). Using M-mode allows ultrasound users to follow the as low as reasonably achievable (ALARA) principle because the intensity of M-mode is less than what is obtained during pulsed-wave Doppler interrogation. M-mode should be the first choice to attain the fetal heart rate because the energy is distributed along the entire wave that is sent into the patient. In contrast, a spectral display should not be used because the energy is only located within the sample gate, which can lead to tissue heating. M-mode does not allow the patient to hear the heartbeat, but the user can explain that it is a safer choice for early pregnancies.

IMPACT OF EQUIPMENT MAINTENANCE ON PATIENT SAFETY

Ultrasound labs must perform routine preventative maintenance on their equipment to make sure that all parameters are within the acceptable standards for ultrasound equipment. It is up to the sonographer to make sure that all parts of the equipment are inspected on a regular basis. Sonographers should make sure that the machine is plugged in to the correct electrical outlets and that the cords do not present a tripping hazard. There are many fundamental pieces of the machine that may be connected to the patient at the same time. The transducer is an integral part of the ultrasound machine and is the component that is always directly on or within the patient. This contact would account for the greatest risk of injury to the patient during an exam. Not only could a damaged transducer degrade the quality of an image, but also a cracked transducer could impart an electrical shock to the patient.

Interactions of Sound and Matter

MEASURING INTENSITY CHANGES

Decibels (dB) are a logarithmic ratio between the amplitude, power, and intensity of the ultrasound beam. They are calculated by dividing the most recent intensity measurement by the original intensity measurement. A positive change in dB indicates that the intensity of the wave is becoming larger or increasing. When there is a +3 dB change, the intensity of the wave is twice as large. A +10 dB change indicates that the intensity is 10 times greater. A negative dB change represents a signal that is becoming weaker or decreasing. For example, a –3 dB change indicates a reduction of the signal by half of the original intensity. If there is a change of –10 dB, it represents a reduction of the original beam by one-tenth.

COMPONENTS OF ATTENUATION

Recall that as a sound beam pass through the body, the intensity is diminished (as are the amplitude and power). Three components contribute to the attenuation of a sound beam: reflection, scattering, and absorption. Reflection occurs if a part of the sound beam is sent back toward the transducer. There are two types of reflection: specular and diffuse. Specular reflection takes place when there is a smooth boundary. This portion of the beam, however, does not return directly back to the transducer, but at an angle. Diffuse reflections take place at a boundary that is not smooth and tends to reflect in various directions known as backscatter. Scattering is the second component of attenuation and occurs when the energy tends to travel in many directions. One cannot predict where scattering will take place. Absorption is the third component of attenuation—this is when the energy of the ultrasound wave is converted to heat.

EFFECT OF DISTANCE ON ATTENUATION

Attenuation is measured in dB and is defined as a decrease in amplitude, power, and intensity as sound travels in the body. In soft tissue, two components that influence attenuation are the distance traveled and the frequency of the ultrasound beam. There is a direct correlation between attenuation and the distance that the sound beam navigates. There is a direct relationship between the frequency of the beam and attenuation. In other words, sound beams that are required to travel a longer distance will demonstrate greater amounts of attenuation and become weaker. Using higher frequencies will also cause greater attenuation of the ultrasound beam. A sound beam that travels a short distance will have a lesser degree of attenuation than a beam that is stronger. Lower frequency transducers will create a beam with less attenuation.

RELATIONSHIP BETWEEN ATTENUATION COEFFICIENT AND FREQUENCY IN SOFT TISSUE

The attenuation coefficient describes how the intensity of the ultrasound beam decreases with regard to the distance and frequency of the ultrasound wave. The attenuation coefficient units are decibels per centimeter (dB/cm). Attenuation occurs because of reflection, scattering, and absorption of the sound beam's energy. Frequency is directly related to scattering and absorption; therefore, frequency is also directly related to the attenuation coefficient. Assuming that the medium in which the ultrasound wave is traveling is soft tissue, the frequency and the attenuation coefficient are directly related. Specifically, the attenuation coefficient is half of the frequency:

$$attenuation\ coefficient = \frac{frequency}{2}$$

If the distance and attenuation coefficient are known, one may determine the total attenuation using the following equation:

$$total\ attenuation = attenuation\ coefficient \times distance$$

RATE OF ATTENUATION IN BONE, LUNG, AND SOFT TISSUE

Attenuation refers to the weakening of sound waves traveling through tissue. As sound travels, there will be a reduction in the intensity of the wave. When comparing attenuation rates of tissue within the body, soft tissue (e.g., liver, spleen, brain, and kidneys) will fall in the middle range. Media with the lowest rate of attenuation are bodily fluids such as urine, amniotic fluid, and blood. Water has no attenuation when examined with low-frequency transducers. Bone tends to absorb a large portion of the ultrasound beam, which allows for a high rate of attenuation when compared to soft tissue. In the lungs, air tends to allow for the absorption of the sound wave; therefore, air is considered to have the highest attenuation rate.

RELATIONSHIP BETWEEN ATTENUATION AND SPEED OF SOUND

Attenuation is the reduction in strength of an ultrasound beam as it passes through the body. It is determined by how far the ultrasound wave travels. More attenuation takes place (i.e., the sound beam loses more strength) with waves that travel greater distances. The frequency of the ultrasound beam also affects how much attenuation takes place. High-frequency sound waves result in greater amounts of attenuation, whereas lower frequency beams will attenuate to a lesser degree. The speed of sound is unrelated and does not factor in when determining how much attenuation a wave will undergo.

Relationship Between Scattering and Frequency

The correlation between scattering and frequency is a direct relationship. Lower frequency sound waves tend to result in less scatter than higher frequency waves, which scatter more. Scattering is a process that can be described as either a random or an organized modification of the direction of the sound beam. An example of organized scatter is Rayleigh scattering. This process tends to alter the direction of the sound wave 360°. Rayleigh scattering also has a direct relationship with the frequency of the sound beam and can be represented by taking the frequency to the fourth power. For example, if the frequency triples, then Rayleigh scattering can be calculated by taking the frequency to the fourth power, shown as follows:

$$3 \times 3 \times 3 \times 3 = 81$$

Relationship Between Penetration Depth and Frequency

Two main items influence the amount of attenuation that a sound wave will sustain. The depth or distance that sound travels in the body is the first item. If a sound beam travels a greater distance, this will result in greater attenuation, which equates to a decrease in intensity of the sound beam. The frequency of the wave is the second item that determines the amount of soft-tissue attenuation. There is more attenuation in sound beams that have a higher frequency; therefore, lower frequency sound will provide less attenuation. Attenuation is directly related to distance and frequency. In order to provide optimal diagnostic images, one should use the highest frequency waves possible and still be able to visualize them at the depth where they are located.

Effects of Density and Speed Increase on Impedance

Impedance is the obstruction of the transmission of sound as it attempts to move through tissue. Impedance is the product of a medium's density and the propagation speed of the medium; therefore, if the density and speed increase, the impedance will also increase. Acoustic impedance is a calculation that has an impact on the amount of reflection that occurs. If two tissue types have the same impedance, then all of the sound will be transmitted. If two tissue types have vastly different impedance rates, then the majority of the sound will be reflected. For example, sonographers cannot easily image an adult brain because very little sound will be transmitted through the skull. If a sonographer is imaging a soft tissue and bone interface, almost all of the sound will be reflected from the bone. In the example of an ultrasound of the adult brain, a low-frequency transducer would have to be used, which will provide images with poor detail.

Relationship Between Impedance and Incidence

Recall that incident intensity is the intensity of a sound beam prior to coming into contact with a boundary. The transmitted intensity is the forward propagation of the intensity of the incident beam after hitting that boundary. Normal incidence is when the incident sound beam comes into contact with the boundary at a 90° angle. Note that a reflection will only occur if the two types of tissue have different impedances; otherwise, transmission occurs. During diagnostic imaging, there is very little difference in the impedance of soft-tissue boundaries; therefore, more than 99% of the incident beam will be transmitted. To summarize, with normal incidence (90°) and identical impedance of the media, all of the incident beam's intensity will be transmitted. Keep in mind that the incident and transmitted intensities must always equal 100%.

HALF-VALUE LAYER THICKNESS

The half-value layer thickness refers to how far sound is transmitted in order for the intensity of the wave to be reduced to half of the original intensity. The half-value layer is also known as the penetration depth or half-boundary layer and describes attenuation. It can be calculated with the following formula:

$$penetration\ depth = \frac{3}{attenuation\ coefficient}$$

Intensity is measured in dB, so it can also be thought of as the distance that the ultrasound beam will travel in tissue to reduce the original intensity by 3 dB. For diagnostic imaging, the range of the half-value layer is 0.25–1.0 cm. This thickness depends on the frequency of the sound as well as the medium it is transmitted in. Half-value layers tend to be smaller for sound traveling at a higher frequency and those tissues that have higher attenuation rates. The half-value layer is greater for lower frequency sound and tissues that have a lower attenuation rate.

RAYLEIGH SCATTERING

Recall that scattering is an erratic, unsystematic diversion of the ultrasound beam in multiple directions. Rayleigh scattering is just one type of scattering, but instead of being erratic, the sound wave is directed in 360° in an organized manner. Rayleigh scattering takes place because the actual size of the target is much smaller than the wavelength of the ultrasound beam. For example, if a sonographer can visualize blood flow in hepatic vessels without color flow Doppler, it is due to Rayleigh scattering. The red blood cells are the target of the ultrasound system, but the image may be misinterpreted because, without color flow, the vessels may appear as if they are clotted. If the user decreases the frequency, then the signal amplitude of what may appear as a clot in the hepatic vessels should be less apparent. Rayleigh scattering is proportional to the frequency to the fourth power.

ECHOGENICITY

Echogenicity refers to the ability of a tissue or structure to produce echoes. It is a very important concept in ultrasound imaging. There are various ways to describe echogenicity based on brightness levels. **Hyperechoic** describes tissues or structures that produce echoes of **high intensity** when compared to adjacent tissue. These tissues will appear brighter than others on the ultrasound image. In contrast, **hypoechoic** describes tissues or structures that produce echoes of **low intensity** when compared to surrounding tissues. They will appear darker on the ultrasound image. Structures that produce **no echoes** at all are referred to as being **anechoic**. Structures that are fluid filled such as the bladder or cysts will produce an anechoic appearance, making them black on ultrasound. Sometimes, there are tissues or structures that produce echoes that are very **similar to those of adjacent tissues**, making them harder to differentiate. These tissues are described as being **isoechoic**.

Tissues or structures with **varying levels of brightness and darkness** are referred to as being **heterogeneous**. Sometimes, these variations in echogenicity can indicate pathology, such as tumors. On the opposite end of the spectrum, there are tissues that display **uniform levels of echogenicity** throughout their entirety and are referred to as **homogeneous**. The brightness remains consistent throughout, without the variations that are seen in heterogeneous structures. Homogeneous echogenicity is typically seen in normal, healthy tissues and can be used as a baseline when assessing tissue characteristics for abnormalities.

Having a thorough understanding of echogenicity is a key skill for a sonographer. Understanding its clinical significance helps determine whether a tissue or structure is normal or abnormal, which improves diagnostic accuracy.

TISSUE DENSITY

Tissue density refers to how concentrated the biological structures within a tissue are. This density has a profound impact on sound waves. For example, a tissue of higher density results in increased attenuation. Bones or calcifications have relatively high densities and therefore may cause shadowing artifacts and affect the image clarity. Higher attenuation weakens sound waves and influences the appearances of structures on the ultrasound image. The resulting image is then poorly visualized.

PENETRATION

The term **penetration** in sonographic imaging refers to the depth that sound waves can travel through tissues. Various structures may be harder to visualize due to their depth—adjusting and optimizing the settings for specific tissues characteristics can help with penetration depth. Abdominal organs such as the liver, pancreas, and kidneys are deep structures that require adequate penetration for sonographic assessment. Lower frequency waves are optimal for deeper penetration. However, there is a trade-off because lower frequencies result in poorer resolution.

DEPTH

Depth is the distance from the ultrasound transducer to the furthest point that structures are being imaged within the body. The depth is a parameter that sonographers can adjust to help visualize structures appearing at different depths within the body. It is important to adjust the depth to match the specific structure that is being imaged, not wasting valuable space on the image. Excessive imaging depth can result in poor temporal resolution. To ensure the acquisition of diagnostically valuable information, there must be a good balance between depth and resolution.

ULTRASOUND LIMITATIONS

As with any imaging modality, ultrasound can face limitations in visualizing certain structures or tissues. Being aware of these limitations will prepare sonographers to deal with potential imaging challenges and help image interpretation. Two of the most common limitations in ultrasound are bones and patient body habitus.

Bone has a high acoustic impedance; therefore, the visualization of bones, or structures beyond bone, with ultrasound is extremely limited. Structures with high density, such as calcifications, can also reduce the quality of ultrasound imaging.

For patients with high tissue thickness (such as those with obesity), there is increased attenuation of ultrasound waves. Therefore, ultrasound imaging in an obese patient can have limited image penetration, which can result in poor image quality. Certain parameters can be adjusted in this case. Although higher frequency transducers are great for resolution and imaging superficial structures, lower frequency transducers allow for better penetration and can help overcome these limitations in patients with thicker tissues.

Imaging Techniques

ESTABLISHED IMAGING PROTOCOLS

Sonographers should be familiar with the established imaging protocols for a range of clinical indications, including abdominal, OB, vascular, cardiac imaging, etc. Each protocol has certain specifications that cover transducer selection, scanning methods, patient preparation and positioning, and anatomical areas needing to be imaged.

It is important to note that these protocols may be modified based on the patient's history and unique clinical indications as well as the request of the referring physician. Different institutions also have their own guidelines when it comes to their protocols. Thus, when performing any ultrasound examination, sonographers should adhere to the rules of their specific institution and confer with the referring physician or radiologist as needed.

ELEMENTS OF ABDOMINAL ULTRASOUND

Patient preparation and positioning: For abdominal ultrasound, patients can be positioned in various ways such as upright, supine, or decubitus. Ultrasound imaging can be significantly impeded by bowel gas. To minimize bowel gas interference, the patient should be instructed to fast for a specified period prior to the examination.

Transducer selection: A low-frequency curvilinear transducer is often used for abdominal imaging. Lower frequency curvilinear transducers are suitable for this type of imaging—they provide deeper penetration and a wider field of view, which are essential for imaging deep abdominal structures such as the liver, kidneys, and pancreas.

Organ-by-organ evaluation: The liver should be evaluated for its size, echogenicity, and contour, and it is assessed for any focal lesions. The gallbladder should be assessed for the presence of any stones, wall thickening, or signs of inflammation. Both kidneys should be comprehensively evaluated for their size; echogenicity; cortical thickness; renal vasculature; and the presence of any stones, cysts, or masses. The pancreas should be visualized to assess for its size; echogenicity; and the presence of any masses, cysts, or dilatation of ducts. The abdominal aorta should be thoroughly evaluated for the presence of aneurysms, thrombi, or other vascular pathologies. The spleen should be evaluated for its size; echogenicity; and the presence of splenic cysts, abscesses, or other pathology. Color and spectral Doppler techniques should also be used as needed to assess for vascular abnormalities such as portal hypertension or stenosis.

Scanning technique: A systematic survey of the entire abdomen should be conducted, using the sagittal and transverse scanning planes to obtain comprehensive views of the abdominal organs and vasculature. All images obtained should be appropriately annotated to facilitate efficient documentation of findings. All measurements, along with a detailed description of any abnormalities, should be reported to the referring physician or radiologist.

ELEMENTS OF OBSTETRIC ULTRASOUND

Patient preparation and positioning: For early pregnancy scans, the patient should be instructed to have a full bladder, which tends to enhance the visualization of the female pelvic structures. Note that fluid-filled structures have a low attenuation rate and therefore can produce acoustic enhancement. The bladder acts as an acoustic window, making it easier and clearer to visualize early pregnancy structures. The patient should be as comfortable as possible, positioned either lying down or in a left lateral decubitus position.

Transducer selection: Before choosing a transducer, the clinical indication and gestational age should be considered. A high-frequency transvaginal transducer is typically the probe of choice in early pregnancy scans (i.e., in the first trimester) because they have great resolution. Conversely, curvilinear transabdominal probes are common for later pregnancy scans (i.e., in the second and third trimesters).

Trimester evaluation: Evaluation of pregnancies via ultrasound can differ depending on the trimester. For example, the first-trimester scan typically involves confirming an intrauterine pregnancy by assessing the presence of a gestational sac, yolk sac, fetal pole, and cardiac activity. The second-trimester scan involves a more detailed anatomical survey such as placenta location and assessing the fetus for any abnormalities. This is known as an anatomy/anomaly scan and typically includes an assessment of various fetal organs such as the brain, spine, abdomen, heart, lungs, and extremities. Certain biometric measurements should also be performed, including fetal abdominal circumference, femur length, head circumference, etc.

Scanning technique: A thorough inspection of the uterus and adnexa should be performed, assessing the gestational sac, embryo/fetus, placenta, amniotic fluid, and maternal anatomy. Transverse and sagittal scanning planes should be used to obtain various views. All findings should be thoroughly documented in the report and promptly communicated to the physician.

GRAYSCALE IMAGING

The most basic form of real-time or grayscale imaging is known as brightness mode. This method is more commonly referred to as B-mode imaging. It was the first grayscale imaging method available. During B-mode, pulses are sent into the body, and, when the signal returns, it appears as a dot on the screen. The amplitude, or strength, of the reflectors will be visualized as dots. Higher amplitudes will appear as bright-white areas on the screen. The areas that return weaker signals will be seen as gray dots on the image display. Even when color mode is used, the underlying image showing the actual anatomy of the patient is represented by grayscale imaging.

MINIMUM TRANSDUCER COMPONENTS NEEDED TO MAKE A GRAYSCALE IMAGE

There are many components of an ultrasound system that are necessary to create an image. In order, the components that are used are the pulser, beam former, receiver, memory, and image display screen. The pulser applies voltages to the transducer in order to excite the active elements within the probe. The pulser functions will take place during transmission of the ultrasound beam. The beam former controls the time delays when phased-array technology is used. The receiver collects the returning signals from objects being imaged so that the data can, as an end result, be viewed on the image display screen. Memory is where the information is kept until it can be displayed on the image display screen.

PARAMETERS INCREASED WHEN AN OPERATOR INCREASES THE OUTPUT POWER

Increasing the output power will have an impact on many parameters. One impact is that the sonographer will be able to penetrate deeper into the body of the patient. Another parameter that is adjusted is the brightness of the image. When the output power is increased, the image becomes brighter throughout the entire display. If the output power is decreased, the overall image becomes darker. Increasing the output power will force the pulser component of the ultrasound machine to increase the amount of voltage that the piezoelectric lead zirconate titanate (PZT) crystals receive in the transducers. This will create stronger pulses that are sent into the tissue, which, in turn, creates an image that is brighter because of the amplified signals. It is important to note that output power is also referred to as acoustic power or output gain.

SOUND IN A VACUUM

Ultrasound users should be aware that sound cannot actually travel through a vacuum. A vacuum does not contain particles that can oscillate and propel the sound. Sound waves actually require a medium to carry the waves. Various types of human tissue are considered to be great media that allow the particles within them to move to help the sound propagate. Recall that during the movement of sound, molecules oscillate to create compressions and rarefactions that change the shape of the molecules. The effects that the tissue (i.e., the media) has on the sound waves are known as acoustic properties. Biologic effects refer to the effects of the sound beam on the biologic tissue.

HIGH CONTRAST

If the image displayed on an ultrasound system has a high amount of contrast, this means that the pixels are either black or white. In ultrasound images that are considered to be high contrast, very few shades of gray are visible. Sonographers should be familiar with the term dynamic range, which controls how the intensity of the signals is transformed into various shades of gray. This will either increase or limit the different shades of gray. For instance, if only black and white shades are created, then there is a narrow dynamic range. A dynamic range that shows many shades of gray would be considered to have a wide dynamic range. These images will be considered to be of low contrast. The dynamic range can be changed on the ultrasound system. If the user believes that the image is grainy, the dynamic range can be increased. If the image is too smooth, the user can decrease the dynamic range.

ADJUSTMENTS TO BETTER VISUALIZE UTERINE FIBROIDS

There are a couple of adjustments that a sonographer can select on the machine in order to better visualize a uterine fibroid. In a transvaginal approach, coded excitation could be used if the machine offers this setting. This technology allows for better penetration when higher frequency transducers are used so that structures in the far field are visualized more readily. This will also improve the image resolution. Another setting that could be used is edge enhance to better delineate the differences in grayscale to make the edges of the fibroid stand out against the normal uterine tissue. Yet another option for sonographers is to choose a different grayscale map altogether. The resolution of the contrast will either be increased or decreased when different selections are made. The user can scroll through the options to determine the best contrast resolution.

PIXEL DENSITY

A pixel refers to all of the tiny boxes that will each have their own gray shade in order to make up a digital image. In order to gain an image with greater resolution, a higher pixel density is required. Pixel density is the number of boxes per inch on the display. A high pixel density will offer better resolution because there will be more pixels found in every inch of the image. This, in turn, requires the pixels to be smaller, which is what is desired when trying to improve the spatial resolution. If an image has a lower number of pixels, the pixels will be larger, so the spatial resolution will not be as great. This is considered to be a low-pixel-density image.

SPATIAL RESOLUTION AND PIXEL DENSITY

Pixel stands for picture element. A pixel is the smallest portion of an image that is in a digital format. For example, a picture taken with a digital camera is made up of thousands of picture elements. Each pixel will consist of one color. Spatial resolution is a term that sonographers are familiar with, and it also applies to other digital technology. Pixel density refers to the number of pixels contained in every inch of an image. The more pixels that an image contains, the higher the spatial resolution will be. A high pixel density will dramatically improve an image whether it is on a digital camera, flat-screen TV, or ultrasound display.

CALCULATING THE NUMBER OF SHADES OF GRAY

A bit has a value equal to either 1 or 0, and it refers to the smallest unit of information that a computer can store. In computer language, there are 8 bits in 1 byte. A bit is the abbreviation for binary digit. For example, to calculate how many shades of gray there are in 4 bits, take 2 to the nth power, where n is the number of bits. This correlates to $2 \times 2 \times 2 \times 2 = 16$. This demonstrates that in 4 bits of memory, there will be 16 different shades of gray. Ultrasound images that contain many shades of gray will offer better contrast resolution.

B-MODE IMAGING

B-mode imaging is also referred to as brightness mode imaging. This refers to a series of dots that are processed by the machine in which the amplitude of the reflector corresponds to a white dot or a gray dot on the image display. The x-axis (horizontal axis) correlates to the depth of the reflector signal that is being returned to the probe. This information is determined by the time of flight. In soft tissue, the depth can be calculated with precision when the time of flight is known. The 13 microsecond (μs) rule also applies when the ultrasound beam travels in soft tissue. It is known that it takes 13 μs for sound to travel 1 cm. If the time of flight is 26 μs, the depth of the object being imaged is 2 cm.

GRAYSCALE ARTIFACTS
MIRROR ARTIFACT

A mirror artifact will always be visualized at a depth greater than that of the actual structure being imaged. It is known as a mirror artifact because a very strong reflector tends to redirect the sound waves as it strikes the mirror. This mirror will appear between the actual object being imaged and the second copy of the structure. The second copy will be equidistant from the reflector as the object, but it will be at a greater depth. This artifact can appear not only in grayscale imaging, but also during color Doppler interrogation. In this case, a second vessel may appear deeper than the actual vessel, but it is actually a mirror artifact. When imaging the abdomen, a common mirror imaging artifact visualized is lung tissue on either side of the diaphragm, which is seen as a bright reflector.

SHADOWING ARTIFACT

Shadowing is visualized when a highly attenuating structure is situated just above this artifact. Shadowing artifacts can often prevent the user from seeing underlying anatomical structures, but they may also serve as a helpful diagnostic indicator during ultrasound exams. A shadowing artifact appears as a hypoechoic or anechoic area deep to the structure that is highly attenuating. Sonographers may notice shadowing posterior to calcifications such as kidney stones and gallstones to aid the radiologist in making a correct diagnosis. The artifact that appears completely different than those characteristics of a shadowing artifact is known as enhancement. In this case, a hyperechoic region appears deep to a structure that is weakly attenuating. Although the appearance of enhancement artifacts is very different, they provide a radiologist with helpful information when discerning tissues.

REFRACTION ARTIFACT

Refraction is the bending of a sound beam when it travels from one medium to another. Two conditions must occur in order for refraction to take place in a clinical setting: (1) There must be an oblique incidence, and (2) the two media must transmit sound at different speeds because refraction cannot take place if they have identical speeds. This is demonstrated in the following diagram:

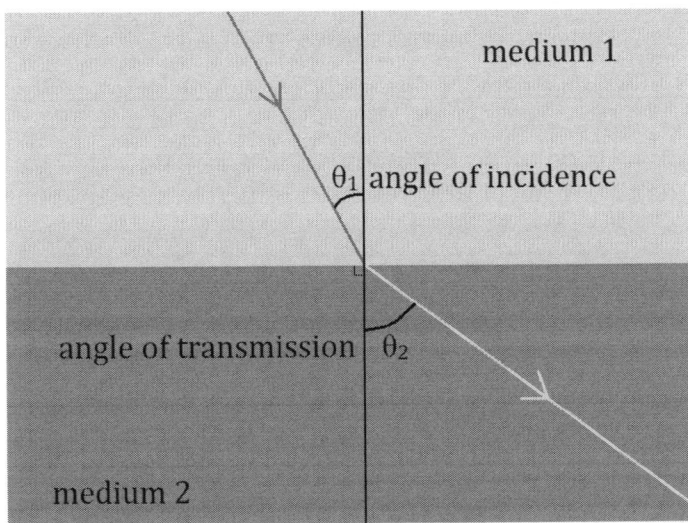

Clinically, an ultrasound beam will only bend slightly at various tissue interfaces. Bone tends to create larger refraction angles because the speed of ultrasound in bone is faster than the speed of ultrasound in soft tissues. Snell's law is used to calculate refraction, and the following equation may be used:

$$\frac{\sin(\theta_2)}{\sin(\theta_1)} = \frac{speed\ in\ medium\ 1}{speed\ in\ medium\ 2}$$

ENHANCEMENT ARTIFACT

While imaging a structure that is fluid filled, for example, a cyst or the gallbladder, the tissue that is visualized posterior to these structures often appears extremely echogenic. The artifact that is the opposite of shadowing is known as an enhancement artifact. These visualized fluid-filled structures are the result of a lower rate of attenuation than the tissue that surrounds them; therefore, structures below them may appear brighter. Shadowing produces a hypoechoic area behind an object that is highly attenuating, and it can prohibit visualization of the structures that extend underneath these structures. Enhancement can be of diagnostic value because radiologists rely on this enhancement artifact to reassure them that a structure is cystic.

Edge Shadow Artifact

A shadow protruding from the edge of a curved structure that is parallel to the axis of the ultrasound beam is referred to as an edge shadow. These are hypoechoic or anechoic structures that may prevent the sonographer from visualizing underlying anatomical structures. These artifacts are created from a decrease in intensity as a sound beam refracts and diverges at the same time after making contact with a curved reflector. These artifacts are often seen when performing an ultrasound of a cyst or during a testicular scan.

Reverberation Artifact

Reverberation artifacts appear as a stepladder and will be in a location that is parallel to the ultrasound beam. Although the first two reflections closest to the probe actually exist, the numerous reflections deeper to them do not and are considered artifacts. These artifacts are created as an ultrasound signal bounces between two strong reflectors that are located parallel to the main axis of the ultrasound beam. These bright reflections resemble a ladder because they contain several "rungs" and are evenly spaced. Another way to describe the appearance of a reverberation artifact is as a set of venetian blinds. These artifacts will always be the same distance from each other. If the distance is 0.5 cm between interfaces, the first reverberation will be 0.5 cm deeper than the object and will be seen at 1 cm. The next artifact will be at 1.5 cm, and the next one will be at 2 cm, until they can no longer be seen on the display.

Lobe Artifact

Lobes refer to unintended echoes that appear outside of the sound beam's main axis. They can negatively affect image quality and diagnostic accuracy. The two types of lobe artifacts are known as side lobes and grating lobes.

Side lobes refer to additional lobes of energy that extend outward from transducers with a single element. In contrast, grating lobes are secondary lobes of energy that result from transducer array elements. Side lobes and grating lobes result in declination of the lateral resolution.

Lateral Resolution Artifact

Lateral resolution artifact is a type of imaging error characterized by the system's inability to differentiate structures that are side by side when the beam is too wide. When the ultrasound waves interact with two structures perpendicular to the ultrasound beam, they display the echoes as being a single structure instead of two distinct points. These structures merge and appear as blurred streaks or smudges.

Axial Resolution Artifact

Axial resolution artifacts are similar to lateral resolution artifacts. However, it is the ultrasound system's inability to accurately differentiate structures that lie one in front of the other, parallel to the sound beam's main axis. A long pulse strikes the two structures, and the system is unable to display the structures as being distinct and separate. As a result, the structures along the axial direction will also merge and appear blurred.

Reject Control

Low-level reflections can be cleaned up by using the reject control on the ultrasound system. On some machines, this may be known as rejection, threshold, or suppression, and it can be used to exclude weakened echoes from appearing on the ultrasound screen. Electronic noise produces low-level reflections; the reject control can be used to reduce this noise. Because every echo must have a set minimum amplitude in order to be displayed, this control determines what that value is so the signals are not processed, thus eliminating the noise.

Ability to Correct Imaging Artifacts

Unintended errors or distortions in ultrasound images are known as artifacts, and they can compromise diagnostic accuracy. Certain artifacts can hide important information, but others can offer insightful diagnostic data. The ability to recognize helpful artifacts and correct the ones that are less valuable is essential to obtaining high-quality ultrasound images.

Imaging artifacts such as acoustic shadowing provide diagnostic information about the presence of high-attenuating structures such as calculi, while acoustic enhancement can confirm the presence of cystic structures and accentuate structures beyond it. However, if the sonographer determines that either of these artifacts is obscuring important details, then certain parameters such as the gain or focal depth can help balance enhancement and reduce shadowing for clearer visualization.

Imaging artifacts such as side lobes and grating lobes can be minimized by processes known as apodization and subdicing. **Apodization** involves changing the intensity of the ultrasound waves to improve beam characteristics, therefore suppressing the off-axis beam lobes. **Subdicing** is a technique that reduces grating lobes by dividing each element (i.e., dicing) into smaller subelements. This helps enhance resolution and mitigate the effects of grating lobes.

Other types of artifacts such as lateral resolution and axial resolution artifacts do not provide diagnostically valuable information because they do not represent the true anatomy at all, by merging two separate structures into one. These types of artifacts require correction. To minimize the effects of lateral resolution artifacts, the sonographer can adjust certain parameters such as the focal depth. Lateral resolution is best where the beam is the narrowest—the focus. To minimize the effects of axial resolution artifacts, a higher frequency transducer can be used since higher frequencies results in shorter pulse durations, which are optimal for axial resolution.

Other types of imaging artifacts include clutter, ghosting, and crosstalk, which all appear in various Doppler imaging modes. Clutter artifact appears on spectral Doppler. Low-frequency, slow-moving signals from the motion of nearby structures are mistakenly displayed on the spectral waveform. Ghosting artifact is like clutter artifact, but it appears on color Doppler. Slow-moving signals from nearby tissue motion can be mistaken for blood flow, and the color appears to "bleed" or extend from the walls of the vessel of interest. The Doppler wall filter is a useful tool that can filter out low-frequency signals and is thus beneficial in correcting clutter and ghosting artifacts. Crosstalk artifact is like mirror image artifact but instead appears on the spectral Doppler waveform. The appearance of identical Doppler waveforms on both sides of the spectral baseline is indicative of crosstalk. Adjusting the angle of insonation minimizes crosstalk artifact in Doppler imaging as well as mirror artifact, which appears on grayscale imaging.

Modify Scanning Technique to Accommodate Reflectors

Optimizing image quality requires an understanding of the behavior of sound waves as they interact with different tissues or structures (reflectors). The scanning technique should be adjusted accordingly.

Based on a reflector's depth, the appropriate transducer frequency should be chosen. Higher frequencies are optimal for reflectors that are more superficial. Higher frequency transducers also provide great resolution. For reflectors that are located deeper, lower frequency transducers are the better choice since they can penetrate deeply. However, the sonographer should know that lower frequencies, although great for penetration, degrade the resolution.

Beam Steering

In ultrasound, beam steering is the manipulation of the direction of the sound beam to visualize different structures. Depending on the type of transducer, beam steering can be achieved either mechanically or electronically.

Mechanical transducers achieve beam steering by physical means. This type of transducer only has one active element, which is physically rotated to mechanically steer the beam in various directions.

Annular-array transducers are also mechanically steered. Other transducer arrays, such as linear sequential and phased arrays as well as curvilinear and vector transducers, accomplish beam steering by electronic means. Sonographers are able to use system controls to adjust this parameter, allowing for the precise imaging of specific anatomical structures.

Electronic beam steering in a phased-array ultrasound system describes the capability of changing the ultrasound beam's direction without requiring physical movement of the transducer. With this tool, sonographers can maximize imaging by viewing anatomical features from various perspectives.

To fully comprehend beam steering in a phased-array system, spiked lines that act as electrical signals are typically illustrated on a diagram. Through the firing of electrical signals that are applied to each piezoelectric element in the transducer, the ultrasound beam can be guided in different directions. Considering the spike line diagram, when the spike lines (i.e., the electrical signals) are arranged straight across in a line—the ultrasound beam is steered straight ahead. However, when there is a slope of the spike lines, the ultrasound beam is steered in different directions. The transducer array's timing or phase shifts can be measured by looking at the slope of the spike lines. When the slope rises from left to right (i.e., the lines become steeper from left to right), this indicates that the electrical signals are steering the ultrasound beam to the right. Conversely, if the spike line slope decreases from left to right (i.e., the lines become shallower from left to right), this indicates that the ultrasound beam is being steered to the left.

EXAMPLES OF APPLYING THE EXTENDED FIELD OF VIEW FUNCTION
VISUALIZING THE ACHILLES TENDON

Many methods are available to obtain an accurate measurement of the Achilles tendon; however, some of these processes tend to be quite invasive. Ultrasound can be used as a noninvasive technique that enables users to obtain accurate measurements of the Achilles tendon. It is a painless, fast, and inexpensive method that can also be used for follow-up studies. Because the Achilles tendon in adults is longer than the face of an ultrasound transducer, many machines have extended field of view or panoramic imaging capabilities. Ultrasound is also sensitive to measure the thickness of the Achilles tendon that does not require extended field of view images, but this information can be useful in cases of tendinopathy. Achilles tendons that have greater thickness measurements tend to be at a greater risk for tendinopathy.

VISUALIZING THE ABDOMINAL AORTA

If the radiologist would like to visualize as much of the abdominal aorta as possible, the sonographer could use the extended field of view control on the ultrasound system. This panoramic image is available on most modern ultrasound equipment, and it replaces the split-screen method of demonstrating objects that are longer than the transducer face. By acquiring various volume data, the system will stitch the information together in order to display one image. This single image will offer clinicians the ability to visualize the entire structure at the same time. This application can be used when interrogating the abdominal aorta, and it may provide additional information regarding the exact location of aneurysms that may be encountered. Often, anatomical structures are enlarged and may be difficult to obtain measurements from. These include the thyroid, testes, musculoskeletal exams, as well as breast lesions.

3D AND 4D IMAGING
OB EXAMS

The two-dimensional (2D) imaging mode is still used to obtain various measurements of the fetus during OB exams; however, three- and four-dimensional (3D and 4D) technology offer even more applications for OB patients. The 3D imaging mode offers one more dimension to the 2D study. The 4D study is real-time 3D, and it offers not only a 3D image, but one that shows the movements of the fetus.

The 3D and 4D imaging modes offer family members a more realistic portrayal of the fetus than 2D imaging. The 4D mode imaging is more than just a lifelike picture of the fetus. Many 4D applications offer improved diagnostic confidence during an OB ultrasound: Echocardiograms, looking at the fetal face for cleft lip/palate deformities, watching the fetus swallow, viewing the fetal spine, checking for skeletal dysplasia, measuring lung volumes, and diagnosing diaphragmatic hernias are just a few examples of what can be studied in greater detail with 4D imaging.

3D Rendering

Postprocessing allows ultrasound users to manage information after it has been stored in the ultrasound system's scan converter. For example, anything that a sonographer does to a frozen image is a postprocessing technique. All postprocessing applications can be undone because the original data are saved. The 3D rendering is one example of a postprocessing technique. The data are required, and the image is either reconstructed on the ultrasound system or it is sent to an offline workstation that is equipped with special software to manipulate and analyze the images. Other examples of postprocessing would be to adjust the gain after an image is frozen or to magnify the image after it has been frozen.

Contrast Imaging

Contrast ultrasound imaging involves the use of contrast agents. These agents are great at improving the visualization of different organs, vessels, and tissues. The enhancement of blood vessels helps delineate their vascularity. The application of contrast imaging in ultrasound is commonly referred to as **contrast-enhanced ultrasound**. This type of ultrasound is primarily used to enhance the visualization of vascular structures, assess blood flow and perfusion, as well as identify any abnormalities. Contrast-enhanced ultrasound can also assist with guiding interventional procedures such as biopsies, ensuring safe and correct needle placement.

Safety Considerations

For safety reasons, sonographers should ensure that they conduct a thorough review of the patient's medical history to identify any contraindications or risk factors. Patients may have allergies to contrast agents, which may result in adverse reactions. Sonographers should be aware of any patient allergies to ensure the safe use of contrast agents in imaging.

The procedure, as well as any benefits or risks, should be explained in detail to the patient. The patient's consent should also be obtained before beginning the contrast-enhanced ultrasound exam. Before, during, and after the exam, the patient should be monitored closely for any signs of complications. By following these guidelines, sonographers ensure a safe and effective use of contrast agents in ultrasound imaging.

Contrast Agents

Microbubble contrast agents are used in patients (either orally or injected) in order to discern abnormal from normal tissues. These agents are used in an ultrasound exam to highlight the visualization of blood flow with respect to the surrounding tissue. Echocardiograms are one type of exam that use contrast agents. There are several specifications that contrast agents must have in order to safely provide a different reflector from those in soft tissue and blood. These gas bubbles must be able to transfer out of capillaries while allowing adequate time for an exam to be performed. Intravenous contrast agents are extensively applied in imaging breast, renal, liver, pancreatic, ovarian, and prostate cancers.

Fusion Imaging

Fusion imaging (also known as hybrid imaging) is a technique that provides sonographers and clinicians with increased diagnostic confidence when following up lesions discovered on previous MRI or CT studies. Fusion imaging also reduces the amount of radiation that a patient is exposed to because ultrasound does not use radiation. Yet another advantage is the greater dynamic monitoring during invasive procedures. Real-time virtual sonography is one example of hybrid imaging that allows grayscale, color Doppler, or the use of contrast harmonics and CT or MRI images to be displayed simultaneously. The CT or MRI images must be sent to the ultrasound system so that the same cross-sectional image can be recreated with sonography. Fusion imaging requires a sensor that is attached to the transducer that will be able to determine the probe location during the scan as well as a transmitter that is attached to the patient.

Measurements
Units Used When Calculating Volume

One of the advantages of sonography is being able to quickly measure organs or other anatomical structures within the body. These measurements are useful in the follow-up treatment of many diseases. These measurements can be added to and displayed on a calculation worksheet for the physician that will be interpreting the results. To calculate the volume of an organ, the sonographer will measure it in three planes using 2D ultrasound. Volume is displayed in any units of length cubed and is calculated by multiplying the length times the width times the height. Organs are typically measured in centimeters; therefore, the volume is in centimeters cubed (cm^3). Three-dimensional ultrasound is also used to calculate the volume of an organ. This method is actually considered to be superior to measurements obtained on 2D images, but it requires more time to perform.

Conversion of MHz to Hz

Sonographers are familiar with the term megahertz (MHz) because diagnostic imaging transducers typically range from 2 to 15 MHz. In the metric system, M stands for mega (megahertz), and the number it equates to is 1,000,000, or 1×10^6. For example, if the transducer being used is an 8 MHz probe, how many hertz is this equal to? This number can be calculated by multiplying 8 times 1,000,000, which gives us 8,000,000 Hz. Another way to convert it is to simply move the decimal point six places to the right. The number 8 can be thought of as 8.0; therefore, moving the decimal six places to the right, add six more zeros to get the result: 8,000,000.

Resolution and Beam Angle

During routine grayscale imaging, axial resolution is superior to lateral and elevational resolution. Axial resolution is the ability to correctly portray two objects (front to back) that are located parallel to the main portion of the ultrasound wave. Axial resolution is not affected by the depth of the reflector, and it relies heavily on the spatial pulse length because shorter pulses create images with better detail. Lateral resolution is how two objects are portrayed when lying next to each other or perpendicular to the ultrasound beam. Elevational resolution attempts to resolve the question of whether the reflectors are within the beam or located above or below it. For instance, when measuring the thickness of the endometrium, the sonographer would want to take the measurement at an angle that is parallel to the beam so that the axial resolution is the most accurate.

Ellipse Feature in OB Ultrasound

After the first trimester, the sonographer may use the ellipse feature to measure the perimeter of the fetal head and abdomen. The user is trying to obtain a circumference measurement when evaluating the fetus. Circumference can be thought of as the perimeter or distance around a circle. Most fetal heads are not circular in shape, but the circumference measurement is used along with other anatomical measurements in order to determine the fetal weight, estimated age of gestation, and the due date. The head circumference can give the clinician important information pertaining to not only the weight of the fetus when combined with other parameters including not only the biparietal diameter, femur length, and abdominal circumference, but also information pertaining to brain development.

Documentation
Picture Archiving and Communications System

A picture archiving and communications system (PACS) allows users of digital imaging to electronically share and archive images so they can be viewed on a network. Clinicians and other medical personnel can also access diagnostic imaging reports because they can be stored on a PACS. PACS has been used to replace film for facilities that have converted to digital imaging systems. This not only saves storage space for the film and chemicals used to process film within imaging departments, but it also allows more than one user to visualize studies at the same time as well as grants instantaneous access to the stored images. If a patient comes into the emergency department (ED) with an abdominal aortic aneurysm, not only can an ED physician view the images, but a surgeon can also see the images in the operating room. Over time, film studies tend to deteriorate, which will not occur with studies that are archived with PACS.

Disadvantages of a PACS

A PACS offers storage and sharing capabilities for facilities that provide imaging services. Whether this facility is part of a hospital or outpatient center, referring physicians and specialists can access the patient's imaging studies along with their reports. This is a huge advantage of having a PACS, but the disadvantages are the initial cost of the system and the equipment required. Because it is a computerized system, it requires an exclusive team of information technology professionals to manage it. Protocols must be in place in case a PACS is not accessible. End-user training is required for all employees and providers that will need access to the PACS. Referring physicians located off site must have the system installed on their computers and must be granted access to use the PACS.

DIGITAL IMAGING AND COMPUTERS IN MEDICINE

The Digital Imaging and Computers in Medicine (DICOM) standard can be thought of as the link between an ultrasound machine (or any other digital imaging system) and a picture archiving and communications system (PACS). DICOM allows for integration of the networks, printing devices, workstations, and PACS that are in use (which are often purchased from multiple vendors). These protocols allow the ultrasound machine to send the images to the PACS network for archiving purposes. In contrast to JPEG images, DICOM images are extremely large—one cannot just load the images onto a computer. DICOM data are not recognized by the Microsoft Windows operating system, so users cannot just double click on an image to load it. A DICOM browser is necessary so that images can be viewed on various computers, workstations, or even a compact disc.

DISC STORAGE

Modern ultrasound machines produce high-resolution images of anatomical structures, but the exams create very large files. Many facilities today archive studies on a PACS, but some prefer to have a backup of the patient's exams. One affordable way that centers may choose to do this is to save the exams on optical media such as laser discs or compact discs. The advantages of these storage devices tend to be that they are economical, they have large capacities, and they will not be erased if exposed to a magnetic field. They do, however, require a browser in order to view the images on a computer. It is also necessary to decide where these discs will be stored so that they can be retrieved, if necessary.

DISADVANTAGES OF STORAGE REQUIRED TO PROCESS FILM

There are disadvantages any time that films must be processed. First, a darkroom is required, which can take up a large amount of space within an imaging department. An adequate supply of film must be on hand. Second, a processor is necessary in conjunction with the darkroom. A processor requires chemicals and periodic maintenance and cleaning. Next, chemicals must be purchased, stored, and refilled when exhausted. Films must be stored, which also takes massive amounts of space. The films must be organized so that they can be found with ease. Artifacts can occur with films, especially if they are not stored under proper conditions (i.e., in the proper temperature and humidity). Processing artifacts can also occur if the chemicals are contaminated or if the processor is not working properly. Some departments have laser film printers, which do not require the use of a darkroom or chemicals, but these films must also be stored under proper conditions.

Capturing Live Clips of Ultrasound Exams

Ultrasound is an imaging modality that relies heavily on the skills of the sonographer. The interpreting physician typically reads the study while reviewing still images. Many years ago, unless an entire exam was videotaped, the ultrasound operator was the only person to see a dynamic study. Modern ultrasound systems offer cine loop storage in which the operator can send short live clips to the interpreting physician. These clips can be stored on the PACS and on CDs so that surgeons can view the exams in real time. This can increase diagnostic confidence during exams that require compression or Valsalva maneuvers, pediatric imaging such as pyloric stenosis studies, and renal exams. Cine loop can also be useful if patients are unable to hold their breath. A sonographer can use cine to capture images in which there is no patient motion in order to freeze an image that could be of diagnostic value.

Ultrasound Transducers

Transducer Components

PIEZOELECTRIC EFFECT

The word **piezoelectric** has Greek and Latin origins. From Greek, *piezo-* means "to press." Electric comes from the Latin *electrum* and means "amber." Amber was used in early electricity studies. Piezoelectric materials such as quartz and tourmaline can be found in nature, but they can also be synthetic/man-made. The piezoelectric material typically seen in transducers is lead zirconate titanate (PZT) because it is readily manufactured.

The piezoelectric effect is the creation of voltage as the result of applied pressure to this piezoelectric substance, deforming the active element. PZT crystals are not naturally piezoelectric; the piezoelectric effect is created when the crystal is subjected to a strong electrical field while being heated to its Curie temperature. As such, the polarized material can become depolarized if the PZT crystal is heated above its Curie temperature.

PZT CRYSTAL

The material in a transducer goes by several names, including the **active element**, **crystal**, and **ceramic**. It is important to be familiar with the various ways of referring to the element. All piezoelectric elements in transducers are shaped like a coin, but they can vary in thickness and material. These factors can be selected by manufacturers to determine the emitting frequency of the transducer.

The diameter of the piezoelectric element does not affect the frequency of the sound wave; however, the thickness of the element does play a part in determining the frequency. The thickness of the PZT element has as inverse relationship with the frequency; therefore, thicker crystals result in lower frequencies, and thinner crystals allow for higher frequencies. For diagnostic probes, the thickness of the active element is usually 0.2–1.0 mm.

There is also a direct relationship between the speed of the sound in an element and the frequency of the pulsed wave. A higher speed through the crystal results in a higher frequency. If the sound wave travels more slowly through the ceramic, the frequency will be lower. This is demonstrated with the following formula:

$$frequency \text{ (MHz)} = \frac{speed \; of \; sound \; in \; PZT \text{ (mm/µs)}}{2 \times thickness \text{ (mm)}}$$

BACKING MATERIAL

Only imaging transducers use backing material. Backing material (also known as the **dampening element**) is made of plastic or epoxy resin and metal powder (typically tungsten filaments). It is located behind the PZT crystal. With similar impedance to the PZT crystal, backing material is efficient in retaining (i.e., absorbing) the energy of the sound. Backing material is used to limit vibrations of the PZT crystal and optimize the axial resolution, which is the ability of the ultrasound system to display structures that are parallel to the sound beam. Shorter spatial pulse lengths and durations help differentiate structures in front of/behind each other. Just as the backing material decreases the vibrations of the PZT crystal upon transmission, the reception of the sound wave is also dampened.

Consequences of using backing material include less conversion of low-level echoes into effective electrical signals, a wide bandwidth, and a lower Q-factor. Without backing material, the PZT crystal will continue to vibrate for a long time once it gets an electronic voltage. An extended duration of the vibrating produces longer pulses, which diminishes the axial resolution.

This is a basic drawing of a transducer in which the backing material is behind the PZT crystal, thus reducing the vibrations to create shorter, pulsed sound waves. The matching layer is the face of the transducer.

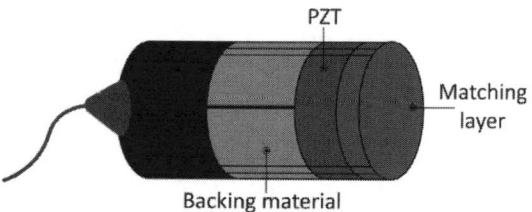

Matching Layer

The matching layer enables the ultrasound energy to make a smooth transition from the probe into the patient's body. At the face of the transducers, the matching layer helps protect the active element. The PZT crystal has an impedance ~20 times higher than soft tissue. Impedance (calculated by multiplying the speed of sound by the density of the medium) influences the reflections produced as sound travels from one medium to another. Without the matching layer, only 20% of the waves would be able to penetrate the skin's boundary. Not only would the sound wave have trouble transmitting through the skin, but the returning echo's intensity would also be reflected.

The matching layer is typically one-fourth the wavelength of the sound. By decreasing the impedance between the PZT crystal and the skin, sound waves are better able to penetrate the skin; however, the matching layer is not enough to get a sufficient signal to and from the body. The impedance between the matching layer and the skin is further reduced through the use of gel.

Reject Function

Rejection is the final process that takes place in the receiver. This function can take place automatically by the ultrasound system, or it can be adjusted by the sonographer. Although the ultrasound machine will automatically reject low-level echoes, the user is able to filter out the remaining echoes depending on if they are diagnostic or meaningful. The reject function can be used in color Doppler and in pulsed-wave Doppler. Some ultrasound manufacturers will have other names for rejection, such as **suppression** or **threshold**.

Transducer Types

LINEAR- AND CONVEX-ARRAY TRANSDUCERS

Arrays are operated in one of two ways: sequencing or phasing; however, there are also differences in how the elements in the transducers are arranged. The elements in **linear transducers** are arranged in a line. The PZT crystals in **convex transducers** are "bowed outward," creating a convex footprint.

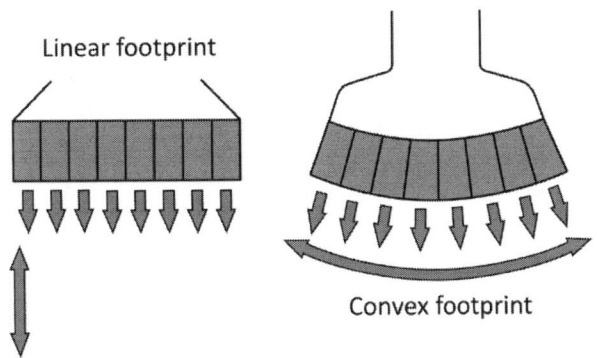

The image above demonstrates the arrangement of PZT crystals sending signals. The linear footprint, on the left, has the signals going straight down into the body. The convex footprint, on the right, shows the bowed-out shape sending waves in different directions outward.

LINEAR-ARRAY TRANSDUCER

Linear sequential array transducers (also referred to as linear switched arrays) usually have a footprint that is slightly larger than the transducers that create fan-shaped images. There are several active crystals (usually 120–250 in number) that are arranged in a straight line across the transducer face. Modern focusing and steering are done electronically, allowing for multiple focus zones. Linear sequential array transducers enable groups of crystals to send signals at the same time, forming the sound beam. When one element in the transducer is damaged, vertical dropout of the image ensues.

Linear sequential arrays are used for various applications. They are useful in imaging shallow structures and small parts, such as the thyroid, breast, and tendons. In addition, linear sequential transducers are useful in imaging vasculature in the neck, arms, and legs. Although most abdominal organs are typically scanned with a curvilinear transducer, superficial structures in the abdomen, such as the gallbladder, can be imaged with a linear sequential transducer.

CONVEX ARRAY

Convex-array transducers, also known as curved- or curvilinear-array transducers, have the elements arranged in a curved line instead of a straight line. Operating like a linear sequential transducer, the PZT crystals (ranging from 120 to 250 in number) in a convex array transducer are activated in groups from one end of the array to the other. The sound beams sent from the crystals are sent in different directions due to the PZT crystals being in an arc shape. Convex-array transducers produce a blunted, sector-shaped image. Using electronic steering and focusing, convex-array transducers achieve dynamic receive focusing, where the signals returning from the transducer to the ultrasound system are slightly delayed. When the PZT crystal is damaged, vertical dropout of the image can occur.

Convex transducers are used for abdominal studies and some pelvic studies. Convex transducers can be used when scanning vasculature at greater depths, such as the renal arteries and veins.

STEERING LINEAR SEQUENTIAL AND CONVEX-ARRAY TRANSDUCERS

Linear sequential transducers and convex-array transducers both use electronic steering. In a convex-array transducer, the PZT crystals are bowed outward. This sends the sound beams out in different directions from the footprint of the transducer. When activated, some, but not all, of the PZT crystals are simultaneously activated.

Unlike convex-array transducers, linear sequential arrays are parallel to each other and typically face straight ahead. Pulses are sent out from the transducers in groups, creating an image that is never wider than the footprint. Firing a small group of active elements instead of a singular element allows for the sound beam to be well defined. The image shape of the linear sequential transducer is rectangular but can become a parallelogram when steering is implemented due to the sloped-pattern phase delays.

LINE DENSITY IN THE NEAR AND FAR FIELDS

Line density is the spacing between the sound beams. Line density is typically described as being either low or high. Low line density occurs when the space between the sound beams is wide, which causes poor spatial resolution. When the line density is low, there are fewer pulses per frame, leading to a high temporal resolution and high frame rate. High line density occurs when the space between the sound beams is thin, which causes great spatial resolution. These tightly packed lines have more pulses per frame, leading to a low temporal resolution and a low frame rate.

Curvilinear-array transducers tend to create sector- or fan-shaped images. As the ultrasound beam disperses further into the body, the line density increases because there is a larger gap between every scan line. As a result of these gaps, the far field demonstrates lower lateral resolution. Linear sequential (switched) probes have a large footprint, and the shape of the image is a rectangle. The crystals in linear sequential transducers are arranged beside each other, and the pulses sent into the body move straight ahead. Because the scan lines travel vertically and are parallel to each other, the line density in the near and far fields will be identical.

PHASED-ARRAY TRANSDUCERS

Transducers with phased-array technology offer focus at different planes and depths. Every PZT crystal is connected to the ultrasound machine's electronic circuit component. Phased-array transducers gain their name through the minute time delays (<1 μs) between singular activation of the crystals. The delay in excitation of crystals is called phasing.

Phased-array transducers allow adjustable focus or even multiple focal zones. Focusing can be optimized regardless of the depth of the anatomical structure being interrogated. Linear phased-array transducers have electronic steering and focusing. Annular phased-array transducers use mechanical steering but electronic focusing.

There are other transducers that use phasing technology that are not phased-array transducers. Examples of these transducers are vector arrays, convex arrays, and linear sequential arrays. These transducers have time delays, but the PZT crystals are excited as a group.

NUMBER OF ACTIVE ELEMENTS USED TO CREATE A BEAM

Modern probes are called **arrays** and contain multiple active elements to create a sound wave. The PZT crystal is usually cut into separate pieces (called **elements**) that are placed beside one another and shaped like thin rectangles. The number of elements can vary considerably depending on the type of transducer, ranging anywhere between 100 and 300. Despite the number of elements a transducer has, all of the elements are activated to create a sound beam. The individual elements each create an individual wavelet. These wavelets then either combine or clash, determining the singular focus and direction of the sound wave.

PHASED-ARRAY IMAGE

A phased-array image is created from small time differences when exciting the PZT crystals. There are two types of phased-array transducers: linear and annular. Both transducers have a fan-/sector-shaped image. Malfunctioning of a PZT element results in dropout of the image. In the linear phased array, damage to the PZT element can result in erratic beam steering and focusing. With the annular phased-array transducer, damage to the PZT crystal will cause horizontal dropout of an image. It is important not to confuse linear phased arrays with linear sequential arrays. While the phased arrays have a sector-shaped image, linear sequential arrays create a rectangular image.

ANNULAR PHASED-ARRAY TRANSDUCERS

Annular phased-array transducers have multiple crystals that are shaped like discs and are arranged in a concentric ring, looking like a target. The inner active elements control focusing at shallower depths. Recall that small-diameter active elements produce beams that are focused at more superficial regions. Crystals with bigger diameters allow for focusing at greater depths. Each ring in an annular phased-array focuses at different depths, each deeper than the one before. The result is an image that is comprised of data from each active element's focal zone. Annular phased-array transducers use mechanical steering since there is a motor to physically move the sound beams in different directions.

Linear Phased-Array Transducers

Linear phased-array transducers are typically compact. The rectangular PZT crystals, ranging from 100 to 300 in number, are usually arranged side by side to create a fan-/sector-shaped image.

Linear phased-array transducers are useful in imaging the heart, brain, and sometimes the abdomen. Due to the small footprint, linear phased arrays allow for imaging in an intercostal space. Phased-array technology enables frame rates to be higher, which is useful when scanning the heart. The beam is focused electronically, which allows for the technologist to add additional focus zones if necessary. The focal depth can be adjusted so that images deeper in the body can be seen in greater detail and resolution.

Steering Phased-Array Transducers

Phased-array transducers use an electronic steering process called **phasing**, hence the name of this type of transducer. Sound beams are transmitted in multiple directions without the use of moving parts like those in mechanical transducers. The PZT crystals are excited at slightly different times (<1 μs), called **phase delays**. These phase delays are used to steer the beam right and left. To visualize the phase delay, imagine a line connecting the electrical signals. A straight line indicates that there is no steering. If there is a rise or fall in the line that connects the electrical signal, then there is steering of the ultrasound beam.

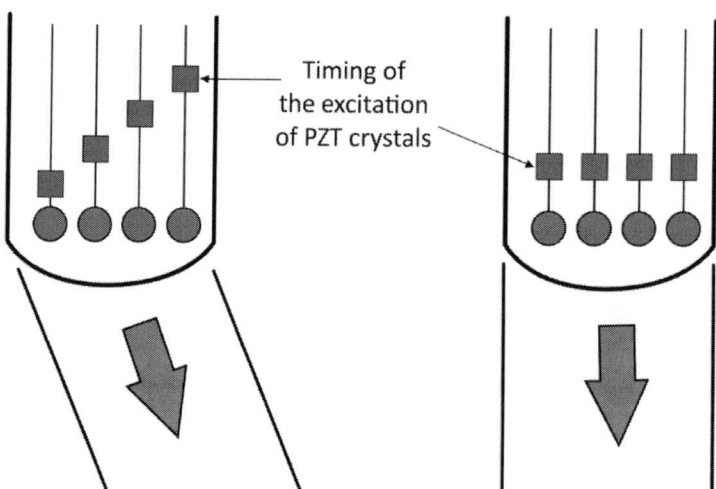

In the image above, the squares represent the electric signals. When the electric signals hit the PZT crystals at the same time (the right image), a straight (unfocused) beam is formed. If the PZT crystals are excited at different times from the electric signals, such as from left to right (the left image), the beam becomes steered to the right.

Two-Dimensional Transducers

Two-dimensional transducers (2D arrays) offer a recent technology that is continuing to be developed and improved. Despite the name, 2D transducers create three- and four-dimensional (3D and 4D) images that have the ability to steer and focus in two dimensions rather than one. These probes contain thousands of piezoelectric elements arranged in what can be compared to the shape of a checkerboard. These beams are electronically focused and steered to obtain volume data. The beam that is transmitted flares outward, catching reflections from structures above and below the presumed imaging plane. A 3D rendering can then be performed on the data collected to create 3D images. This 3D technique is postprocessing as the computer-generated images are manipulated. This technology is used in OB ultrasound as well as diagnostic imaging for various diseases and disorders on nonpregnant populations.

EFFECTS ON SLICE THICKNESS AND CONTRAST WITH 2D ARRAY TRANSDUCERS

Slice thickness can also be known as **elevational resolution**. Slice thickness provides resolution of structures side to side, parallel to the ultrasound beam, and above and below the imaging plane. Two-dimensional array transducer crystals typically have a disc shape, contributing to the best elevational resolution in the focal zone. The height of the circle, from the cross section of the disc-shaped crystal, indicates the beam width. In phased-array, linear-array, and convex-array transducers, the slice thickness is not affected by a narrowed beam. In 2D array transducers, the thousands of PZT crystals across the footprint allow for an extremely thin slice of a sound beam. This thin slice enables better contrast resolution because the beam is smaller than the structure being interrogated. Contrast resolution is augmented due to diminished volume averaging.

IMAGING AND NONIMAGING TRANSDUCERS

Imaging transducers transform electronic signals into sound waves with short durations and pulses. This is achieved using backing materials to limit the amount of ringing. Consequently, the use of backing material decreases the sensitivity of small, reflected echoes. Dampening material produces a wide bandwidth and low Q-factor as a result of the shorter, dampened pulse.

Nonimaging transducers do not use backing material, thus creating continuous waves or pulses with long durations and length. The lack of ringing creates a narrow bandwidth with increased sensitivity to the small, reflected echoes. The higher sensitivity gives continuous-wave transducers a higher Q-factor.

The Q-factor and pulse length have a direct relationship. Longer (i.e., increased) pulses have a high Q-factor, while shorter (i.e., decreased) pulses have a low Q-factor.

Transducer Selection

ADVANTAGES AND DISADVANTAGES OF SMALL-FOOTPRINT TRANSDUCERS

An advantage of transducers with small footprints is that they can be used to scan tight spaces, such as between the ribs (intercostal spaces). A linear phased array is one example of a probe that has a small footprint that touches the skin. It is easier to acquire intercostal images with a linear phased array because the transducer footprint can send sound waves between the ribs. A disadvantage of linear phased-array transducers is that the beam quickly splays apart in the far field, so the lateral resolution offered by these transducers tends to be reduced. This diversion occurs at the region of depth that is two times the length from the face of the transducer.

PENETRATING HIGHLY ATTENUATING TISSUE MORE READILY

Attenuation is the reduction of the intensity of a sound beam as it travels through a medium. Some areas of the body tend to attenuate the sound beam more than others. The lungs and bones tend to have high attenuation because the sound wave becomes scattered, reflected, or absorbed. To allow the ultrasound beam to better penetrate tissue, especially when visualizing organs deeper within the body, the sonographer should decrease the frequency.

Frequency and attenuation have a direct relationship: Higher frequencies attenuate more, while lower frequencies attenuate less; however, although lower frequencies allow for visualization of deeper organs, the detail and spatial resolution of the organs themselves will decrease. Higher frequencies, despite attenuating more, have better detail and greater spatial resolution. As sonographers, it is important to find the balance between great resolution and clear visualization of the organs.

CHOOSING A TRANSDUCER TO MAXIMIZE FIELD OF VIEW

In order to obtain the largest possible field of view in the near and far fields, a sonographer would choose a convex-array transducer. These are also known as curvilinear or curved-array transducers.

The image display from a linear sequential probe is in the shape of a rectangle due to the arrangement of the active elements. The elements form a straight line that directs the pulses in front. The image display from a convex-array transducer, however, is a sector shape that is blunted at the top. The bowed shape at the top of the image directly correlates with the curved shape of the transducer. Because these images do not form a sharp peak at the top, they tend to allow for a wider field of view in the near field and the far field.

TRANSDUCER USED FOR PELVIC EXAMS

Endocavity transducers offer better spatial resolution because of their proximity to the female organs. During a transvaginal or endovaginal ultrasound, the transducer is placed inside the vagina, which allows for excellent image quality. The transducers that are used during a transvaginal ultrasound have high frequency compared to the lower frequency transducers used during a transabdominal exam. This not only allows for better image quality when looking at the various pelvic organs and regions, but it is also easier for operators to obtain Doppler measurements. The bladder is emptied during a transvaginal study, which offers patients relief because transabdominal scanning while the patient's bladder is full is extremely uncomfortable. Transvaginal scanning may also be used in first-trimester OB scans because structures are better visualized due to the close proximity to the transducer. For pelvic exams, clinicians may prefer a transabdominal and a transvaginal approach for a complete workup.

IMPACT OF FREQUENCY ON TRANSDUCER SELECTION

Transducers are created with various thicknesses of PZT crystals in order to provide users with an option to select transducers with different frequencies. When imaging organs at a greater depth, such as the ovaries, a probe with a lower frequency should be used. Recall that frequency and attenuation have a direct relationship, where an increase in frequency results in an increase in attenuation. Less attenuation provides for more image depth, while high frequencies allow for higher resolution images of the organ.

Transducer Assessment and Adjustment

RELATIONSHIP BETWEEN FREQUENCY AND SPEED OF SOUND

Frequency, in regard to sound, is the number of complete cycles that occur in a second. The frequency of the pulsed wave cannot be changed while using a basic ultrasound system and transducer.

The speed of sound through a particular medium is measured in units of distance over time. The speed of sound through a medium is also known as the **propagation speed**. The propagation speed is determined by the medium. All sound travels at the same frequency through a specific medium. In soft tissue, sound usually travels between 550 and 4,000 m/s. The propagation speed has a direct relationship with the stiffness of and an inverse relationship with the density of the medium. Stiffness may also be called the **bulk modulus**.

Although the speed of sound in a medium is not affected by frequency, it can be calculated with frequency and wavelength, as follows:

$$speed \text{ (m/s)} = frequency \text{ (Hz)} \times wavelength \text{ (m)}$$

RELATIONSHIP BETWEEN ELECTRIC AND ACOUSTIC FREQUENCY

The frequency of ultrasound transducers relies on how the active element is activated. It can either be determined by continuous- or pulsed-wave principles. Pulsed-wave ultrasound will send short electrical impulses that travel from the system to excite the piezoelectric lead zirconate titanate (PZT) element in the probe. In contrast, continuous-wave ultrasound transducers tend to steadily induce an electrical impulse that activates the probe's active element. In this case, the electrical frequency determines the acoustic frequency. For example, if the electrical frequency (voltage) is 12 MHz, the acoustic frequency of the sound beam would also be equal to 12 MHz.

Fundamental Frequency and Harmonic Frequency

The fundamental frequency is the actual frequency that is being imparted from the ultrasound transducer and passed into the patient. It is also known as the **transmitted frequency**. The ultrasound beam can become altered, however, causing examinations that are not diagnostic. Modern ultrasound systems offer harmonic imaging to help increase diagnostic confidence in those difficult studies. Harmonic frequencies are created in the tissues during transmission along the beam's main axis. When this occurs, the sound wave is less distorted, improving the quality of the diagnostic scan. The harmonic frequency is two times higher than the fundamental (transmitted) frequency. Tissue and contrast harmonics are two examples of the types of harmonic ultrasound in use today.

Two waves constructively interfering adds the amplitudes but maintains the frequency.

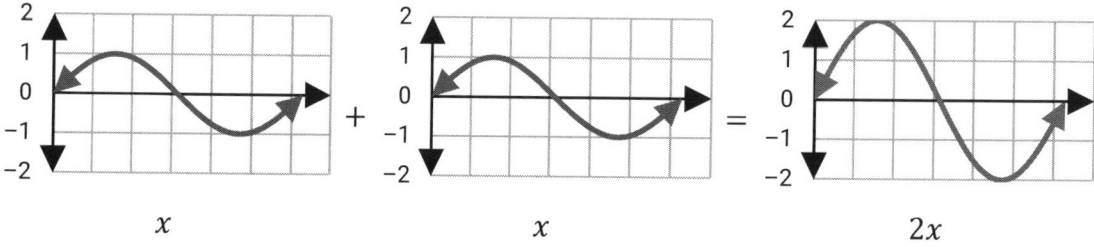

Relationship Between Frequency and Wavelength

Wavelength is the distance or length of one cycle. Wavelength is displayed in any unit of distance. The usual range in diagnostic ultrasound is 0.1–0.8 mm. Wavelength is determined by the source of the sound and the medium through which it is traveling. Although the wavelength cannot be controlled by the sonographer (since the source and medium cannot be changed), it can be calculated by the frequency and propagation speed. Wavelength and frequency have an inverse relationship, so an increase in frequency equals a decrease in wavelength. Conversely, a decrease in frequency equals an increase in wavelength, calculated as follows:

$$wavelength \text{ (mm)} = \frac{1.54 \text{ mm}/\mu s}{frequency \text{ (MHz)}}$$

Relationship Between Frequency and Bandwidth

Bandwidth (or broadband) is the range of frequencies in a singular pulse. Bandwidth can be determined by subtracting the lowest possible frequency from the highest available frequency. For example, if the main frequency (also known as the resonant frequency) is 10 MHz, the range of frequencies transmitted may be adjusted to a frequency between 8 and 12 MHz. The bandwidth can be found via the following equation:

$$12 \text{ MHz} - 8 \text{ MHz} = 4 \text{ MHz}$$

Because imaging transducers can produce many frequencies, they tend to have a wide bandwidth. The use of backing material also produces a wide bandwidth. The shorter the pulse, the higher the number of frequencies contained in the ultrasound pulse.

Frequency and bandwidth can determine the quality factor (Q-factor), which is the main frequency divided by the bandwidth. Imaging probes have a low Q-factor, while continuous-wave transducers have a high Q-factor. The Q-factor is inversely related to the bandwidth.

FOCUSING TECHNIQUES FOR ULTRASOUND TRANSDUCERS

Focusing improves the resolution of an ultrasound image by creating a narrow sound beam. There are various techniques used to focus an ultrasound beam.

External focusing using a lens is one way to improve the lateral resolution. This is an example of fixed focusing (the conventional method) in which a lens embedded in front of the active element and provides a narrow beam in the region of focus. A more common method of fixed focusing that does not need a lens is internal focusing. This form of focusing includes a crystal that has a curved shape, but it also results in a tapered ultrasound beam. Electronic focusing via phased-array technology allows the sonographer to adjust the focus. This technology allows the PZT crystals to send out pulses at different times. Certain return reflections are postponed so that they do not all return to the probe at the same time. This phasing allows for signals to be returned constantly, which allows focusing at all depths. This is only available on probes that have many PZT crystals.

ULTRASOUND IMAGE SHAPES

Sonographers should be aware of the image shapes that certain transducers portray. Phased-array transducers create sector-shaped images. Convex transducers produce blunted sector-shaped images. Linear sequential transducers typically create rectangular images that can become parallelograms when steered. Vector transducers produce trapezoidal images.

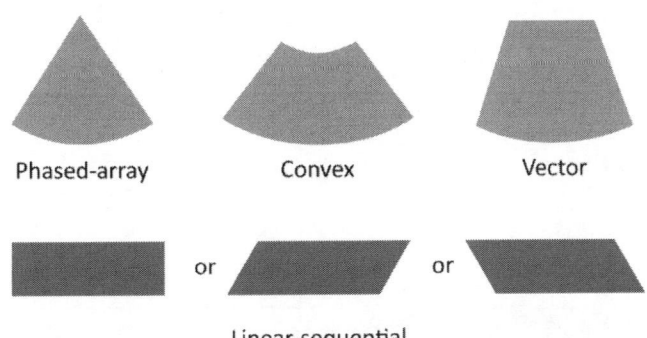

The convex sector top is curved, while the vector transducer top is straight (horizontal). The bottoms of the convex, vector, and phased-array transducers are all curved convex.

Optimizing Sonographic Images

Focus

The **focal point** is also known as the focus or the middle of the focal zone. The focal point is the pinnacle of an ultrasound beam at which point it has been tapered (i.e., narrowed) as much as possible. The width of the ultrasound beam at the focus is half the diameter of the probe. The focal point is the region that offers the best possible image resolution because the beam is the narrowest there. The region around the focus is known as the focal zone, which includes a portion of the near and far fields that are on either side of the focal point. Sonographers should always keep the focal point at the level of the structure of interest. The focus can be adjusted quickly and easily so that the resolution is optimal at that level.

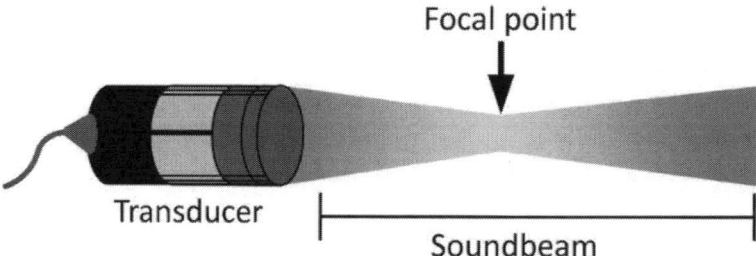

For example, consider a disc-shaped transducer with a diameter of 10 mm that emits a continuous-wave (CW) sound beam. Since the width of the ultrasound beam at its focal point is half the diameter of the transducer diameter, the width of the focal point is 5 mm.

FOCAL ZONE

The **focal zone** of an ultrasound beam is the section that surrounds the focal point. Because the focal zone is a more generalized area than the actual focal point, it is located in the near and far zones of the ultrasound beam. The focal zone is divided equally so that half of it is within the near zone and half is in the far zone. It is recognized that the diameter of the ultrasound wave is narrow in the focal zone, so structures imaged are more reliable than those visualized at other scanning depths. This in turn results in better resolution; however, the focal point is where the beam diameter is tapered the most, so the best resolution is located there.

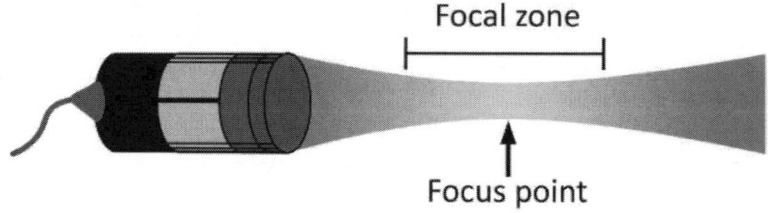

FRAUNHOFER ZONE

The **Fraunhofer zone** is also referred to as the far zone or **far field**. It is the area of the sound beam located distal to the focal point. The focal point marks the beginning of the Fraunhofer zone, which continues diverging. At two focal depths, the diameter of the sound beam in the Fraunhofer zone is the same as the diameter of the transducer. At depths beyond two focal depths, the sound beam diameter exceeds the diameter of the transducer face.

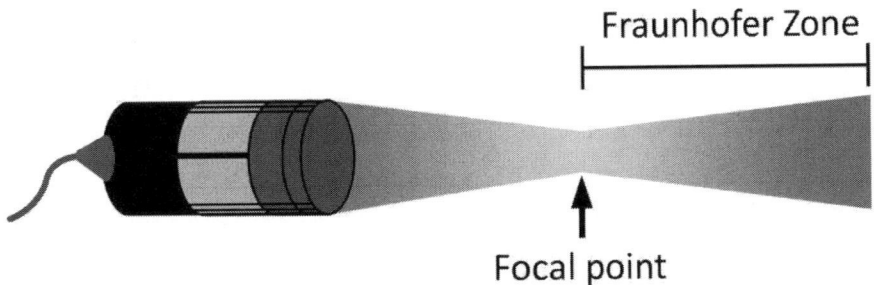

For example, if the transducer face is 6 mm, and the focal depth is 4 cm long, then what is the diameter of the sound beam at a depth of 8 cm? Since a depth of 8 cm is two focal depths (4 cm × 2), the diameter of the sound beam is 6 mm.

FRESNEL ZONE

The **Fresnel zone** (aka the **near field** or near zone) is the area located between the transducer and the focal point. When the sound beam exits the transducer, the beam gradually tapers as it gets closer to the focal point. The length of the Fresnel zone is also known as the focal depth.

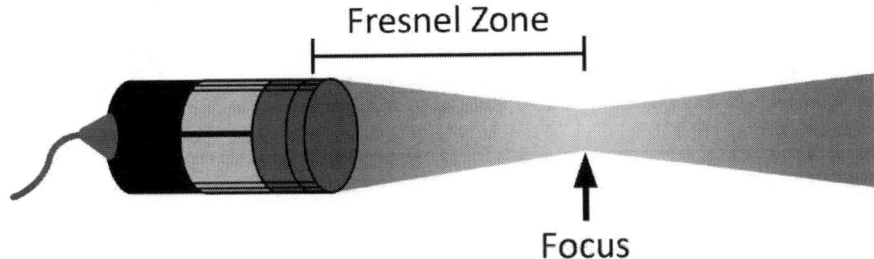

For example, if the focal point is at a depth of 5 cm, then the length of the Fresnel zone is 5 cm because it is the distance between the transducer and the focal point.

EFFECTS OF FOCUSING ON THE ULTRASOUND BEAM

When a sonographer applies focusing during an exam, many changes take place within the ultrasound beam. When the ultrasound beam is focused, the beam diameter beyond the focal point widens. Focusing improves the lateral resolution in the Fresnel zone while degrading the lateral resolution in the Fraunhofer zone. The size of the focal zone is reduced with better lateral resolution because the beam is narrower. Since the focal point has moved closer to the transducer, the Fresnel length is reduced. Meanwhile, the beam diameter in the Fresnel length and focal zone narrows.

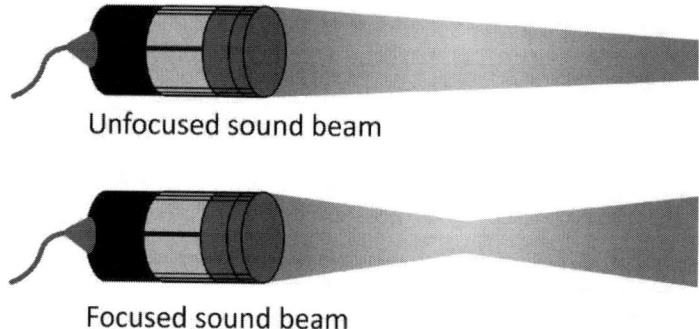

Unfocused sound beam

Focused sound beam

The lower beam is focused. Observe the narrowed beam diameter in the near field and focal point, the decreased Fresnel zone length, the widened sound beam in the Fraunhofer zone, and the smaller focal point.

EFFECT OF USING MULTIPLE FOCAL POINTS ON THE TEMPORAL RESOLUTION AND FRAME RATE

The frame rate is the ultrasound machine's ability to store numerous frames per second. The frame rate is dependent on the sound beam's speed in the structure that it is imaging (soft tissue is considered to be at 1.54 km/s) and the depth of the imaging. The frame rate is typically measured in hertz (Hz), with units of images per second.

Temporal resolution is the ability to precisely position closely spaced events (i.e., movement) from instant to instant. "Good" temporal resolution is when the system is able to produce many frames per second. "Bad" temporal resolution is only being able to produce a few frames per second. The temporal resolution is determined by the frame rate. Higher frame rates yield a higher temporal resolution. Lower frame rates yield a lower temporal resolution. The temporal resolution, like the frame rate, is also measured in Hz.

If a sonographer applies multiple focal zones during an exam, the temporal resolution degrades since this action tends to decrease the frame rate. When compared to using just one focal zone, each additional focal zone requires the system to produce more pulses throughout each scan line, which, in turn, increases the time necessary to produce a single image. This will, however, improve the lateral resolution to more accurately display the reflectors because the beam is tighter within the focal regions. It is up to the sonographer to decide which type of resolution will better aid in providing a correct diagnosis.

EFFECT OF USING MULTIPLE FOCAL POINTS ON LATERAL RESOLUTION

The lateral resolution is improved with sound beams that are narrower. The shape of the ultrasound beam tends to change according to its depth. The lateral resolution tends to be improved at depths in which the sound beam is narrow. This depth is at the focus, and when multiple focal points are used, the beam becomes tapered over a greater imaging depth, which greatly enhances the accuracy of the images produced. Although the lateral resolution is improved when multiple focal zones are used, the temporal resolution tends to decline because more time is necessary to produce the image.

USE OF DYNAMIC APERTURE WITH PHASED-ARRAY TECHNOLOGY

Dynamic aperture is when the focus changes throughout echo reception to maintain a constant focal width, thus optimizing the lateral resolution. Focusing narrows a beam within the focal zone. Without dynamic aperture, the lateral resolution suffers as the beam diverges in the far field. The diameter of the PZT crystals (i.e., the active elements) can aid in determining if the focus will be deep or shallow. If the focus is shallow, the diameter of the PZT crystal is small. In contrast, a diameter that is bigger will create a deeper focus. With dynamic aperture technology, the number of active elements activated can differ from time to time. This keeps the ultrasound beam narrow, improving the lateral resolution for reflectors located at more positions within the ultrasound beam.

RELATIONSHIP BETWEEN THE FOCAL DEPTH AND THE DIAMETER OF THE TRANSDUCER

Focal depth refers to the distance from the transducer to the focus of the sound beam. With a fixed focus transducer, the focal depth is dependent on the transducer's diameter and the frequency of sound. The transducer's diameter and the focal depth are directly related. If the transducer has a larger diameter, the focal depth will be deeper. If the transducer has a smaller diameter, the focal depth will be shallower. As an example, there are two transducers of different diameters, one with an 8 mm diameter and the other with a 10 mm diameter. Given that the two transducers are otherwise identical (including the frequency of the sound), the 10 mm diameter transducer will have a deeper focus. Larger diameter transducers create deeper foci. This shows a direct relationship.

RELATIONSHIP BETWEEN FREQUENCY AND FOCAL DEPTH

The focal depth is determined by the transducer diameter and the frequency of the sound. Frequency and focal depth are directly related: increased frequency creates an increased (i.e., deeper) focal depth. To allow better visualization at a shallower depth, ultrasound machine manufacturers have created PZT crystals that are small in diameter but high in frequency.

FOCUSING USING A LINEAR PHASED-ARRAY TRANSDUCER

When a sonographer is using a linear phased-array transducer, the beam former will contain a curved pattern that will allow focusing during an exam. To visualize focusing in a linear phased array, imagine a line connecting the electrical signals. If these electrical spikes form a straight line, the ultrasound beam is not focused. When the spikes are in a curved formation, the beam is focused. The active elements located on the lateral portion of the transducer are fired earlier than those near the middle to help focus the beam. The focus can also be steered along with focusing deeper (if the height of the curve is not very high), or it can be at a more superficial location (if the height of the curve is more prominent). To determine if the focus is being steered, an imaginary line may be drawn between the two outer spikes. If it is a straight line, there is no steering being used. The ultrasound beam may be directed to the right or to the left.

Resolution

AXIAL RESOLUTION

Resolution refers to how precisely an object is being portrayed during a scan. The **axial resolution** determines how close two structures can be to still be portrayed as two separate reflectors on the ultrasound display. The axial resolution is measured in distance, typically in millimeters. The image quality and accuracy are represented with smaller axial distances. In diagnostic ultrasound, the measurements of axial resolution typically lie in the 0.1 to 1 mm range. The smaller the axial resolution, the better. Shorter pulses and brief pulse durations will enhance the axial resolution. Axial resolution is superior to lateral resolution because the pulse lengths are shorter than the width of the beam. Axial resolution is also known as longitudinal, range, radial, and depth resolution.

BOOSTING AXIAL RESOLUTION

Short pulse lengths improve the axial (i.e., longitudinal, range, radial, depth) resolution. Shorter pulses are established by using a transducer that offers a higher frequency and backing material. Diagnostic imaging transducers contain backing material that limits the amount of ringing in a pulse. As manufacturers have reduced the number of cycles per pulse to one to three, the only way the sonographer can improve the axial resolution is by increasing the frequency, which causes more attenuation and less penetration.

LOW-QUALITY-FACTOR TRANSDUCERS

Low-quality-factor (low-Q-factor) transducers are used for diagnostic pulsed-wave (PW) ultrasound because they offer improved axial resolution. Low-Q-factor transducers contain backing material, which controls the amount of ringing that takes place. By restricting the amount of ringing, shorter pulses are created. Shorter pulses will designate better axial resolution and, therefore, improved image quality. The fact that the pulses are shorter with better axial resolution means that most of the ultrasound beam's energy will dissipate after the first couple of oscillations. Another advantage of low-Q-factor transducers is their ability to offer multiple frequencies because of their wide bandwidth. Axial resolution is the kind that offers the most accurate image in modern transducers and imaging systems. Recall that the accuracy of the axial resolution is not affected by the depth of the image, whereas the elevational and lateral resolution are.

CALCULATING AXIAL RESOLUTION

The axial resolution is equal to half of the spatial pulse length. The following formula can be used to calculate it:

$$\text{axial resolution (mm)} = \frac{\text{spatial pulse length (mm)}}{2}$$

For example, using a 3.5 MHz transducer with a pulse length of 6 mm:

$$\text{axial resolution (mm)} = \frac{6}{2} = 3 \text{ mm}$$

Depending on the available information, the axial resolution may also be calculated by the following formula:

$$\text{axial resolution (mm)} = \frac{\text{wavelength (mm)} \times \text{number of cycles in the pulse}}{2}$$

To determine the axial resolution in soft tissue:

$$\text{axial resolution (mm)} = \frac{0.77 \times \text{number of cycles in the pulse}}{\text{frequency (Hz)}}$$

Remember: when the axial resolution is calculated to be a lower number, there will be better image quality because the pulses are short.

FOCAL ZONES

The axial resolution identifies reflectors that are parallel to the ultrasound wave, and it is determined by the pulse length and duration of the pulse. If more focal zones are added, the pulse length will become longer, degrading the axial resolution. Shorter pulses demonstrate better axial resolution. If the sonographer increases the number of focal zones, there will be better lateral resolution, but the width of the beam will narrow.

LATERAL RESOLUTION

Lateral resolution allows a sonographer to visualize two distinct reflectors when they are perpendicular to the sound beam (i.e., beside each other). This type of resolution determines how close two structures can be to each other and still be visualized as two separate objects on the ultrasound display. The units of lateral resolution can be any form of a distance measurement. Values that are smaller indicate finer detail and the ability to image tinier objects. The narrowest part of the beam (i.e., the focus) is where the lateral resolution will be optimal. Lateral resolution is also known as angular, azimuthal, and transverse resolution.

BEAM WIDTH

Ultrasound beams that demonstrate better lateral resolution tend to be the narrowest ones. If two objects are positioned adjacent to each other at a distance that is smaller than the beam diameter, only one structure will be visualized during the exam. The lateral resolution is controlled by the diameter of the ultrasound beam; thus, the best way to improve the lateral resolution is to focus the beam. Recall that the ultrasound beam changes in size and shape with depth, so the lateral resolution also varies with the depth of the beam. The lateral resolution is equal to the beam width:

$$\text{lateral resolution (mm)} = \text{beam width (mm)}$$

IMPACT OF TRANSDUCER FREQUENCY TYPE ON THE FAR-FIELD LATERAL RESOLUTION

Because the lateral resolution is best when the beam is the narrowest, the lateral resolution at the focal point proves to be the best; however, when using high-frequency transducers, the ultrasound beam will be narrower overall than those created with a low-frequency probe. The beam profile depicts that when a high-frequency transducer is used, it reveals less expansion of the beam in the far field (i.e., the Fraunhofer zone). Beams with lower frequencies tend to diverge more in the far field, which results in poorer lateral resolution in comparison. See the section above on the relationship between the frequency and the focal depth.

LINEAR SEQUENTIAL TRANSDUCER

Linear sequential (i.e., switched) transducers are the best choice for small-parts ultrasound exams. The design of the probe, which is long and narrow, allows for easier skin contact of the area being interrogated. This is useful because these regions of the body are often more difficult to reach. The shape that results from this probe is rectangular, which is the most appropriate shape because sector images provide a wide field of view in the far field that is not necessary with these types of exams. While the lateral resolution changes with the scanning depth, these probes have better lateral resolution in the far field than do others due to having higher frequencies. Of course, the lateral resolution is the best at the focal point where the beam is the absolute narrowest, so the best way to optimize the lateral resolution is to use the highest number of focal zones.

ELEVATIONAL RESOLUTION

Elevational resolution is determined by the thickness of the imaging plane. Elevational resolution is the ability to accurately portray structures lying above or below the assumed imaging plane. The slice thickness is also known as the section thickness or partial-volume artifact. The ultrasound beam is not a uniform shape; rather, it varies with depth and takes the shape of an hourglass. Because of this shape, some echoes may be included in the return signal, but they are located either above or below the ultrasound beam. Blood vessels or cysts may appear filled in, rather than anechoic, due to the partial-volume artifact, which occurs when the slice thickness is larger than the size of the structure.

IMPROVING ELEVATIONAL RESOLUTION

Recall that elevational resolution relates to how accurately an object is being imaged when it is perpendicular to the ultrasound beam. The elevational resolution is regulated by the thickness that is in a perpendicular direction when compared to the direction of the ultrasound wave. If the slice thickness is greater than the actual imaging beam, then the elevational resolution will deteriorate and any structures that are located above or below the beam will be visualized in the image. A 1.5-dimensional (1.5D) array probe will provide improved elevational resolution because of the arrangement of the PZT crystals in the vertical and horizontal planes. This will allow focusing to occur in the plane that controls the thickness of the ultrasound beam. Because there is an indirect relationship to slice thickness and elevational resolution, a thinner slice will provide better elevational resolution.

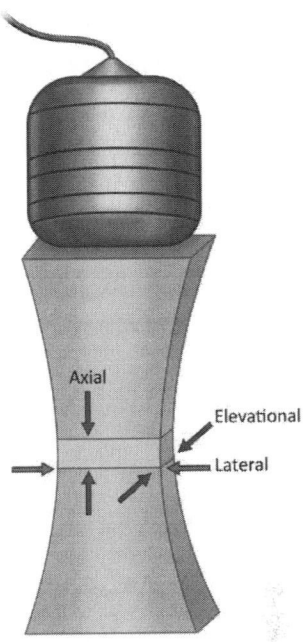

PARTIAL-VOLUME IMAGING ARTIFACT

If a radiologist cannot definitively determine if a cyst-like structure is indeed a cyst, the elevational resolution may be the culprit, exhibiting a partial-volume imaging artifact. Elevational resolution refers to the slice thickness of the ultrasound beam. If the slice thickness of a beam is particularly thick at a certain depth during a scan, the echoes that are returned will correspond to the soft tissues that are located on either side of the cyst.

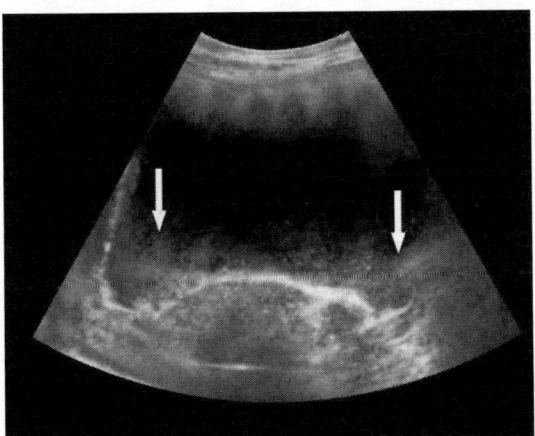

This creates an illusion that the cyst-like structure is filled in, and the radiologist may not be able to determine that it is, indeed, a cyst. A thinner slice will accurately display a fluid-filled structure whether that structure is a cyst or a blood vessel. When a sonographer chooses a matrix-array transducer, the PZT crystals are arranged vertically and laterally, allowing for electronic focusing in both directions. Using a 1.5D transducer will result in a beam that has improved elevational resolution.

TEMPORAL RESOLUTION

Temporal resolution is the ability to accurately image a moving structure. It is dependent on the frame rate: a higher frame rate indicates a better temporal resolution. A higher temporal resolution will more accurately portray the location of a structure from one second to the next. The temporal resolution is considered optimal when there are several frames per second. One of the most common steps performed to increase the temporal resolution is to decrease the depth during an ultrasound exam. A structure that is located deeper in the body will require a greater time of flight because the system is transmitting the pulses into the body and then back to the transducer to be processed. This additional time will decrease the frame rate and the temporal resolution. If the user needs to increase the temporal resolution, the scanning depth should always remain as shallow as possible so there is less time required to process a signal.

OPERATOR CONTROLS THAT AFFECT THE FRAME RATE

The frame rate is the ultrasound machine's ability to create multiple frames per second. A sonographer can adjust the imaging depth and the number of pulses per frame to impact the frame rate. The more detailed the images are, the longer it takes to produce them, thus decreasing the frame rate. For example, if the sonographer decreases the depth (i.e., more superficial), there is less detail in the image, yielding a higher frame rate. If a system is imaging a structure that is deep in the body, the frame rate will be lower. Changes that the sonographer can make to alter the number of pulses sent into the body (e.g., line density) are changing the number of focal zones, adjusting the field of view (i.e., the sector size), and producing a smaller color box.

When the field of view is smaller, fewer pulses are necessary to create the image, which takes less time. The frame rate (i.e., the temporal resolution) is inversely proportional to the sector size of the image. In addition, reducing the number of foci may also improve the temporal resolution. Decreasing the imaging depth increases the frame rate because less go-return time is required since the reflectors are located at a shallow depth.

The frame rate is comparable to Wi-Fi speeds. If there are multiple functions going on at once (e.g., streaming, downloading, browsing, etc.), the Wi-Fi speed will decrease. The ultrasound machine running at an increased depth, color Doppler, and PW Doppler, with multiple foci, will slow the frame rate down.

MULTIPLE FOCAL ZONES

Modern imaging systems have the capability to operate while using multiple focal zones. Using multiple foci will greatly improve the detail of an image, but users must balance the detail with the time required for the study. If a sonographer is looking at an object using a single focus, the temporal resolution will be superior because the frame rate is higher. If additional focal zones are added, not only are more pulses required, but extra pulses are also needed in each scan line. This degrades the temporal resolution because the frame rate is slower. A multifocal sound beam will greatly improve the lateral resolution of an image because the beam is narrowed over many depths, but the temporal resolution will suffer due to the increased number of pulses per frame.

Magnification

READ MAGNIFICATION

Magnification allows users to zoom in on or increase the size of a region of interest. The type of magnification that is performed after an image has already been stored in the scan converter is read magnification. Read magnification is a postprocessing function because it can enlarge an image that has been frozen, but the spatial resolution tends to stay the same because the zoomed-in image still contains the same number of pixels as the original image. The image is not reconstructed by the system; the pixels are just larger than they were in the first image. This function has no effect on the frame rate (thereby, the temporal resolution) because the image will be located at the same depth as the original information. Because the spatial resolution is not any better than the original image, this is not the preferred method of magnification.

Read magnification is comparable to zooming in on a picture after it was taken. This can show very pixelated images because the quality of the photo was set when the picture was captured.

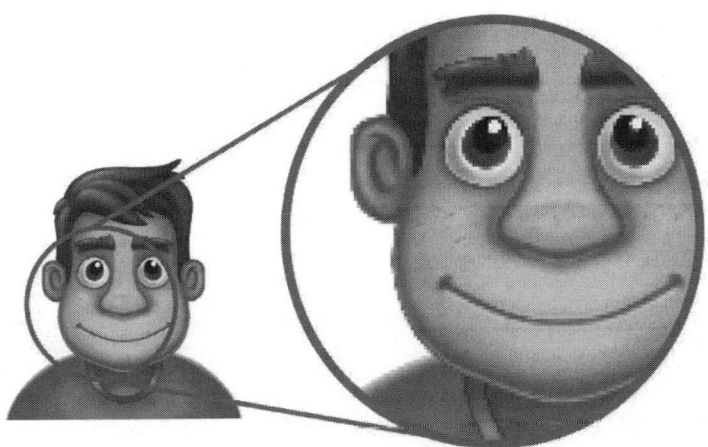

WRITE MAGNIFICATION

The type of magnification that is preferred due to improved spatial resolution is write magnification. It takes place before the data are stored in the scan converter. The area identified in the region of interest is rescanned and old data are ignored to obtain new information. This type of zoom increases the number of pixels when compared to the first image, which automatically increases the amount of spatial resolution. Thus, this magnification process is the preferred method to zoom an image. Because it is completed before the data are stored in the scan converter, it is a preprocessing technique. Once rescanned, the temporal resolution may be improved if the new image is shallower than the original data.

Imagine zooming in to the region of interest on your camera before snapping the picture. The quality of the image would be better than capturing a picture and zooming in afterward.

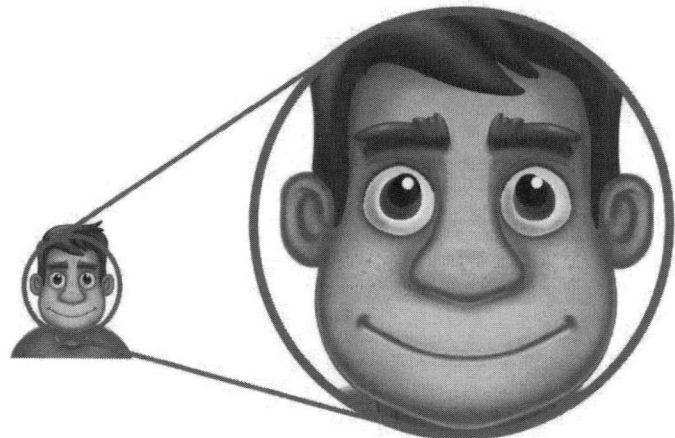

The image on the left shows the region of interest to zoom in to before capturing a picture, which produces a similar effect to write magnification.

Brightness

OVERALL GAIN

There are two adjustments that a sonographer can make to increase or decrease image brightness: output power and overall gain.

Output power strengthens the sound pulse sent by the transducer into the body. Because the sent pulsed wave is more powerful, the returning echoes are more powerful as well, allowing for a brighter image.

Overall gain is also referred to as receiver gain or the amplification of the ultrasound beam. This control affects the ultrasound image by amplifying the returning echoes.

Sonographers should always keep the output power as low as reasonably achievable (ALARA). They must strive to decrease the exposure of sound waves to their patients, when possible.

CHANGING THE OVERALL RECEIVER GAIN

When a sonographer changes the overall gain on an ultrasound system, it amplifies or decreases the returning echoes. This action takes place in the receiver and has a uniform effect on the image by changing the strength of the voltages that the probe has produced. If the receiver gain is increased, a brighter image will appear throughout the entire image. If the gain is decreased, the overall image becomes darker. Unlike output power, if the gain is increased, the signal-to-noise ratio is not changed. An increase in output power will enhance the signal-to-noise ratio.

SAFELY MAKING THE ENTIRE IMAGE BRIGHTER

Sonographers should always keep the ALARA principle in mind during all diagnostic imaging exams. This principle is practiced to reduce the possibility of adverse effects (i.e., bioeffects) during an ultrasound exam. A sonographer may make an entire image brighter by increasing the output power, but this will also increase the exposure to the patient. If output power is increased, more voltage is applied to the transducer, which increases the strength of the pulse sent into the body. A safer alternative to increase the brightness of the entire image is to increase the gain, which does not expose the patient to more powerful voltages: it just amplifies the returning echoes.

SAFELY MAKING THE ENTIRE IMAGE DARKER

The output power or overall gain can be adjusted. If the entire image is too bright, to darken it, the sonographer should decrease the output power before the receiver gain to darken the image. This will result in a lower exposure of strong sound beams.

TIME GAIN COMPENSATION (TGC)

Attenuation is the reduction of intensity of the ultrasound beam as it passes through tissue. Attenuation increases as the beam travels deeper in the body. Echoes that return from a shallower location in the body tend to be stronger than echoes that are deeper. For the sonographer to compensate for attenuation within tissues, the time gain compensation (TGC) or depth gain compensation can be adjusted. This control will typically be slide pods that can be adjusted. Each level represents different depths within the body. The overall goal of TGC is to create an image that demonstrates uniform brightness from the top of the display to the bottom.

REFLECTOR DEPTH

Sonographers can visualize the depth of every reflector because there will be a scale on one side of the image that correlates to how deep the reflectors are in the body. Every dot typically represents 1 cm but can be adjusted by the sonographer. For example, if echoes are too bright at 4 cm from the surface, the sonographer can adjust for the increased echogenicity of the structure by finding the TGC slide pod that correlates to that location and move the slider to the user's left (or toward the right of the ultrasound system). TGC can be used in conjunction with receiver gain (i.e., amplification) to provide an image with consistent brightness throughout.

MEASUREMENT UNITS

Amplification refers to the brightness of an ultrasound signal. Amplification can be measured in decibels (dB). Compensation is a type of amplification, so it is also measured in dB. Amplification is the first process that takes place in the receiver. It will differentiate the strength of the beam as it enters and exits the receiver of the ultrasound system. The normal range for amplification of an image ranges from 60 to 100 dB. Changing only the amplification is not enough to create an image with the same level of brightness throughout. The user must also consider adjusting the compensation, which is the second process in the receiver and can be used in conjunction with amplification to create an image with uniform brightness.

Receiver Functions

The receiver gathers the signals that have been sent into the body that are returned to the transducer to display them on the screen. Five functions take place in the receiver, but they must be completed in the correct order so that images can be displayed: (1) amplification, which increases the size of the signals that are returned; (2) compensation, which adjusts for attenuation that the sound beam encounters as it propagates deeper into the body; (3) compression, which allows the human eye to differentiate between various gray shades to determine which one allows more useful information to be extracted from the image; (4) demodulation, which cannot be adjusted by the system (it has no effect on the actual image—rather, it rectifies the negative voltages); and (5) reject, which affects only low-level echoes on the display.

TGC Curve

A TGC curve has an x-axis as well as a y-axis. The horizontal, or x, axis represents how much compensation is necessary for the depth of the object being imaged (the y-axis). The top of the y-axis represents the patient's skin, and, as it moves down, it refers to tissues that are located deeper in the body. The near gain is located superficially near the skin's surface. At this location, the structures being imaged need very little TGC because not much attenuation occurs. The slope is the middle portion of the TGC curve, where more compensation is necessary because of the greater depths. The knee is located at the distal portion of the slope and demonstrates where the most compensation will occur. The region of far gain is distal to the knee at an ever-greater depth, which also indicates that the greatest amount of compensation has been offered by the machine.

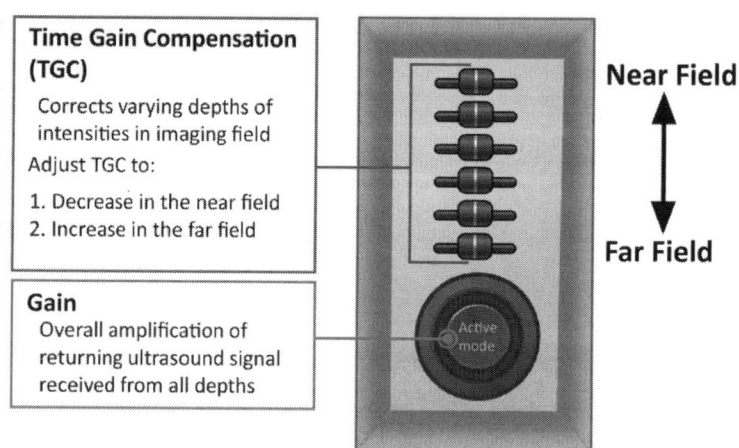

Depth

EQUATION TO CALCULATE THE DEPTH OF AN OBJECT

Ultrasound systems can determine the depth of an object by calculating the time of flight. This time refers to having the transducer send out a pulse, and once the reflector has been identified, the signal is returned to the transducer. Depth can be calculated with the equation $d = \frac{ct}{2}$, where d is the depth, c is the speed of sound in soft tissue, and t is the time of flight.

13 MICROSECOND (µs) RULE

Ultrasound machines are designed to calculate the speed of the ultrasound wave in soft tissue as 1.54 mm/µs. The time of flight refers to the time it takes for a pulse to leave the transducer, hit a reflector, and return to the transducer. For every centimeter of depth the pulse goes into the body, 13 µs have passed. Using this rule, if a target is 2 cm deep, the time of flight will be twice as long, equating to 26 µs. If the time of flight is 39 µs, the depth of the reflector will be 3 cm. Sonographers should be aware of the reflector depth and the total distance traveled. For example, if a question states that the time of flight was 13 µs, and it is asked what the total distance traveled is, the answer would be 2 cm. At 13 µs, the depth to the reflector would only be 1 cm, but the total distance would be 2 cm because the sound beam must travel another 1 cm back to the transducer.

EFFECT OF THE PRF ON IMAGING DEPTH AND RANGE AMBIGUITY

Range ambiguity is an imaging error in which the echoes have not yet been returned to the transducer before the next pulse is transmitted. If the PRF is too high while scanning a structure deep in the body, range ambiguity may occur. If this happens, the system will incorrectly place the received reflections closer to the probe than their actual depth. PRF represents the number of pulses sent into the body every second, and it is presented in units of hertz (Hz). The normal range of PRF in imaging systems is 1,000 to 10,000 Hz. If a sonographer increases the imaging depth, the system automatically decreases the PRF to avoid range ambiguity. In other words, the PRF is inversely related to the imaging depth; therefore, if the scan depth is twice as deep, the ultrasound system will automatically reduce the PRF by half.

SPATIAL PULSE LENGTH

The spatial pulse length has units of distance and describes how long a pulse is from its beginning to its end. The normal value of the spatial pulse length in diagnostic ultrasound ranges from 0.1 to 1.0 mm. The pulse length depends on the sound source and the medium, but it cannot be adjusted by the ultrasound user. The scanning depth has no effect on the spatial pulse length. Operators should be aware that shorter pulse lengths produce images that are more truthful. Short pulse lengths are created when a decrease in the number of cycles is contained within the pulse. The wavelength is also determined by the sound source and the medium; therefore, if shorter wavelengths are present, then shorter pulses are created.

Duty Factor

Duty factor is the percentage or fraction of time that a system is transmitting sound. The duty factor is calculated by the following equation:

$$\text{duty factor} = \frac{\text{pulse duration}}{\text{PRP}} \times 100$$

Duty factor is a calculation that has no units; rather, it will be expressed as a percentage. The ranges of duty factor for clinical imaging are from 0.002 to 0.005 or from 0.2% to 0.5%. These ranges of diagnostic ultrasound indicate that a small percentage of time is spent transmitting a pulse and a large percentage of time is used for listening. For CW systems, the duty factor is 1, or 100%, because a signal is always being sent, but of course an image cannot be created because there are no signals being received. A system with a duty factor of 0% means that a transducer is not being used.

PULSE REPETITION FREQUENCY (PRF)

The pulse repetition frequency (PRF) is the number of pulses sent into the body in 1 second. The duty factor and the PRF are both affected by the imaging depth and will have a direct relationship with each other. The PRF is inversely related to the depth of the object being studied, as is the duty factor. As the depth decreases, the PRF increases because new pulses are constantly being sent because the listening time is reduced. If the depth increases, the PRF decreases (as will the duty factor) because there is more listening time, so the return time is greater. If the PRF increases, the duty factor also increases because the amount of time the system is "on," or transmitting a pulse, increases.

RELATIONSHIP BETWEEN THE PULSE REPETITION PERIOD (PRP) AND THE IMAGING DEPTH

The pulse repetition period (PRP) consists of the time that the pulse is on (i.e., send) and the time it is off (i.e., receive) as pulses are sent out of the transducer. There is a direct relationship between the scanning depth and the PRP. If a sonographer is attempting to scan an object located deep in the body, there will be more listening (i.e., receive) time and a lower pulse repetition frequency (PRF). If the reflector being examined happens to be shallower, the PRP is shorter because the listening time is decreased. Sonographers can change the imaging depth with a control on the ultrasound system. The PRP and PRF are reciprocals of each other and have an inverse relationship.

DETERMINING PRP AND PRF

The PRF and PRP are parameters that can be changed when the imaging depth is modified. The PRF and PRP are not determined by the periods or frequency of the sound wave. Because the PRF and PRP have an inverse relationship, the effect that the scanning depth has on them is also twofold: (1) The PRF and the scanning depth are inversely related. As the scanning depth increases, the PRF will automatically decrease. (2) The PRP and the scanning depth have a direct relationship—as the scanning depth increases, the PRP will also increase because there will be more listening time involved. The relationships between PRF and PRP are shown via the following equations:

$$\text{PRF} = \frac{1}{\text{PRP}} \qquad \text{PRP} = \frac{1}{\text{PRF}} \qquad \text{PRF} \times \text{PRP} = 1$$

The 13 microsecond (μs) rule states that each centimeter (cm) of depth in the body is 13 μs. In soft tissue, the PRP can be calculated as follows:

$$\text{PRP (μs)} = \text{imaging depth (cm)} \times 13\,\frac{\mu s}{cm}$$

For a depth of 8 cm, the PRP is 104 μs (8 × 13 μs).

In soft tissue, the PRF can be found via the following equation:

$$\text{PRF (Hz)} = \frac{77{,}000\ \text{cm/s}}{\text{imaging depth (cm)}}$$

The 77,000 cm/s is due to the speed of sound in soft tissue, 1,540 m/s or 154,000 cm/s. Because the sound wave would need to travel back to the transducer, the total depth that the sound wave would reach in 1 second would be 77,000 cm.

PRF, PRP, AND SHALLOW IMAGING

Recall that the PRF and the PRP are inversely related, so if the PRF is low, the PRP should be high. At a shallower depth, there is a shorter listening time and a shorter PRP. At a deeper depth, there is a longer listening time with a longer PRF.

Harmonic Imaging

ORIGIN OF TISSUE HARMONICS

Tissue harmonics are not emitted from the transducer but are produced when the sound beam interacts with tissues that are deeper in the body in a nonlinear fashion (i.e., sound waves traveling faster through compressions and slower through rarefactions) during transmission. Tissue harmonics do not occur when the scanning depth is shallow. The transmitted sound beams must be strong: weak sound waves will not produce any tissue harmonics at all. Sound beams that are somewhat strong will only produce a small amount of harmonics. With strong beams, the harmonics are created within the main line of the ultrasound wave. Tissue harmonics will only emerge from this main axis and will create very few imaging errors because of the strength of the beam. Beams that are most likely to create harmonics are the least likely to create artifacts.

FUNDAMENTAL AND HARMONIC FREQUENCIES

The fundamental frequency is the frequency of the ultrasound beam produced by the transducer and imparted into the patient. For example, if a 6 MHz transducer is selected, 6 MHz will be the fundamental frequency.

Harmonic imaging corrects the malformation of the ultrasound wave that may take place when the fundamental frequency is used. If the sound beam is distorted, a diagnostic exam may not be possible. The harmonic frequency will be two times larger than the fundamental frequency. For example, if the fundamental frequency is 6 MHz, then the harmonic frequency is 12 MHz. An ultrasound beam that is created with harmonic frequencies will not undergo as much distortion and is less likely to produce images with artifact. When harmonics are used, a strong signal is required, and the signals are created along the main axis of the sound wave.

IMAGING THE GALLBLADDER

The gallbladder is an organ that is subject to image artifact during an ultrasound. It can be difficult to discern if reflectors visualized within it are real. Tissue harmonics is a concept that has helped clinicians and operators gain diagnostic confidence because it tends to eliminate some signals that are not pathological. Harmonic frequencies allow the sonographer to scan patients at higher frequencies, which will not only improve the axial resolution, but will also improve the lateral resolution. The lateral resolution tends to improve because the wave is narrower (higher frequency beams produce a narrower beam). Imaging gallbladders with harmonic ultrasound improves the signal-to-noise ratio, enhances visualization of structures deeper in the body, and eliminates reverberation artifacts, which can mimic sludge within the gallbladder.

M-Mode

M-mode ultrasound refers to motion mode, horizontal lines that represent the changing depth of the reflective surfaces. M-mode offers information pertaining to time, which is represented by the x-axis. As the reflectors move across the screen, they are visualized as the activity is taking place at that specific instant. As the structures move from left to right across the screen, they may shift up or down. This demonstrates whether the object is moving toward or away from the transducer. The y-axis represents the depth of the objects that are in the path of the ultrasound beam. Amplitude is also reflected because some objects will have stronger returning signals than others.

INTERPRETING THE DISPLAY FROM M-MODE

Motion mode (M-mode) is represented by an x-axis and a y-axis. The x-axis is the horizontal portion of the display, which equates to time. The vertical axis is the y-axis, and it correlates to the depth of the reflectors. The go-return time is a way to calculate the depth of the reflector. A higher go-return time correlates to structures that are deeper in the body, and smaller go-return values are the result of signals that are shallower. Moving from right to left, if the tracing moves up, this indicates that the object is closer to the probe. A line that is moving down means that it is moving away from the probe. If the line is a horizontal tracing, it means that the reflector is not in motion. The go-return time is also known as the time of flight.

Using M-Mode

Regarding A-mode (amplification), B-mode (brightness), or M-mode (motion), the only one that offers information pertaining to time is M-mode. M-mode is illustrated by bumpy lines that tend to roll across the monitor from left to right. It is used predominantly in echocardiography or to obtain a heart rate during an obstetrical exam. M-mode is advantageous because it allows greater temporal resolution, so even structures that are moving rapidly can be accurately measured and recorded. The data are obtained from a single line of sight, which allows the user to change the location if necessary. Sometimes this can create erroneous measurements if the single line is not perpendicular to a structure.

Additional Imaging Techniques and Concepts

Compression and Dynamic Range

Compression is a parameter on the ultrasound system that allows a sonographer to change the number of shades of gray that are available to produce an image that is appealing to the user's eyes. The purpose of this feature is to produce an image that contains as much data as possible to make a diagnosis without being particularly dark or overly gray.

The dynamic range is a ratio between the largest and the smallest of intensities that can accurately be displayed by the ultrasound system. The units of dynamic range are decibels (dB). If an ultrasound system produces an image that displays numerous shades of gray (i.e., more information), that image would be considered to have a wide dynamic range. An image with numerous shades of gray is of low contrast. On the other hand, if the system produces an image with a narrow dynamic range, this results in a high-contrast image.

When compressed, the largest signal remains the largest and the smallest signal remains the smallest. The range of signals within is reduced. Compression is sonographer adjustable.

Spatial Compounding

Spatial compounding is a technology that involves a single stationary transducer acquiring multiple imaging angles and combining them into one image. Steering is done from the center of the ultrasound beam and from the right and left sides of the transducer. The resolution is greatly improved when spatial compounding is used because more data are obtained and combined. Spatial compounding is generated at a higher quality with higher frame rates. It will, however, degrade the temporal resolution because more processing is required, and the frame rate tends to slow down.

Spatial compounding is useful for reducing speckle and shadowing artifacts in exams such as musculoskeletal, thyroid, vascular, and breast ultrasounds. Speckle artifacts are created when the ultrasound beam is scattered after interacting with various tissues. Noise that results from speckle artifacts will make the image appear grainy, but spatial compounding improves the signal-to-noise ratio, helping to eliminate some of the noise. Spatial compounding may also suppress the amount of shadowing that is apparent in an image. This is corrected because a single transducer (a phased array) can steer the frames from multiple directions and many angles will be perpendicular to the structures, decreasing the amount of shadowing.

Persistence

Persistence (temporal averaging or temporal compounding) is a method that can be used during grayscale or color Doppler imaging. By overlapping information obtained from older frames onto images more recently obtained, the machine can produce an ultrasound image with greater detail that has less noise, is smoother, and has a higher signal-to-noise ratio. If the signal-to-noise ratio is high, the ultrasound machine effectively suppresses noise. Although the image detail improves with the use of persistence, the temporal resolution is degraded because of the additional processing. This makes imaging structures that are moving rapidly very difficult because there will be a lag as the temporal resolution is decreased. Persistence is best used with structures that demonstrate slow motion.

Spatial compounding averages multiple frames obtained by steering the sound beams in different directions for different imaging angles, whereas persistence uses images from the same view.

Improve Color on Doppler Images

Persistence is an averaging technique that will combine images from older frames with those of newer data. In grayscale imaging, persistence can be used to smooth out an image or reduce the amount of noise present. Persistence is also found to be useful in color Doppler imaging especially if the vessels to be visualized are deeper in the body, to identify vessels that contain slow-moving blood, or if there is an obstruction of a vessel. Smaller vessels can also be identified more readily than with methods that do not implement persistence. The temporal resolution is often decreased when persistence is applied to an image.

Frequency Compounding

Frequency compounding is a method used to reduce the amount of speckle in an ultrasound image. Ultrasound images are filled with speckle, but it is important that a reduction takes place to discern objects that demonstrate low contrast. Targets that are smaller may not be visualized if the amount of speckle is not reduced. Frequency compounding is an averaging method that tends to take the speckle patterns of multiple images into consideration to reduce the noise and speckle artifact that are present.

Reflected waves are subdivided into smaller ranges of frequency. An image is obtained from the smaller ranges of frequencies and combined into a single image. When combined, the noise level is reduced.

Edge Enhancement

If a sonographer wants to improve the image sharpness, edge enhancement can be applied. This is a technique that allows better delineation of the border of structures by sharpening the edges of a mass. Often, it is difficult to discern the differences in tissue types. By raising the image contrast at the interface of these tissues, it will enhance the change that may not be as obvious without edge enhancement. At the boundary between two or more tissue types, various shades of gray are displayed, and edge enhancement will produce edges that are more reflective to help the mass stand out against normal liver tissue, for example. Edge enhancement makes small bright and dark highlights appear to have more defined edges.

Coded Excitation

Coded excitation allows for multiple transmission foci, separation of harmonic echo bandwidth from the transmitted pulse bandwidth, increased penetration, reduction of speckle with improved contrast resolution, and grayscale imaging of blood flow. Penetration and resolution are two important factors when considering the quality of an ultrasound image. Higher resolution is obtained using short pulses during an ultrasound exam. This does, however, increase the chance of bioeffects in the patient. Coded excitation uses a series of pulses and gaps instead of a single driving pulse. This also tends to keep the intensity of the signal well within the limit deemed safe for patients. This is only necessary on high-frequency transducers, such as those used for transvaginal studies. With better penetration and increased resolution in the far field, fibroids can be easier to correctly diagnose.

Doppler Imaging

General Principles

PRF

RANGE AMBIGUITY AND HIGH PRF

Range ambiguity is when the exact location of movement cannot be determined. Recall that range ambiguity artifact (also known as range specificity or range resolution) is typically seen in CW Doppler. When using PW Doppler, range ambiguity is seen when a sample volume is used to determine the exact location in which a velocity measurement should be obtained.

The PRF can be controlled by the "scale" knob on the ultrasound machine. If the PRF is set too high for the depth of the reflector being interrogated, range ambiguity will exist because the system will be directed to send out pulses before the earlier pulses have been returned. If the echoes are not returned in the order that they are transmitted, the system will incorrectly determine the depth of the object being scanned. In this case, aliasing will occur, which can be corrected by increasing the scale.

MAXIMIZE COLOR DOPPLER VISUALIZATION

Color Doppler is often used when assessing the vascular system. If the ultrasound machine is not picking up color with color Doppler, the sonographer can adjust the PRF (via the "scale" button or knob) and increase the color gain. Decreasing the PRF parameter helps to detect blood that is flowing more slowly due to the lower Doppler shifts. A PRF scale that is set lower will enable the system to recognize red blood cells that are moving more slowly because more time is allowed from one pulse to the next. This step will increase the sensitivity of the color Doppler application. Other parameters that can be changed to improve color Doppler sensitivity to low flow would be to increase the Doppler gain and decrease the value of the wall filter.

NYQUIST LIMIT

The Nyquist limit is a term that applies to color Doppler as well as PW Doppler. The Nyquist limit (Nyquist frequency) is the upper extent to a measurable Doppler shift (frequency) that can exist without demonstrating aliasing. The Nyquist limit can be calculated using the following equation:

$$\text{Nyquist limit} = \frac{\text{PRF}}{2}$$

The imaging depth and the transducer's fundamental frequency are not necessary to solve aliasing. If the frequency is higher than the Nyquist limit with PW Doppler, aliasing may occur because the sampling rate is too low.

Types of Spectral Analysis

Spectral analysis is a technique used during PW Doppler ultrasound to provide information pertaining to the various velocities obtained in the blood vessel or organ being scanned. Blood does not travel in the same direction or speed, even when contained in the same sample volume. The spectral analysis window will allow clinicians to examine how the frequency shifts are dispersed within the Doppler signal. Two types of spectral analysis are used: the fast Fourier transform (FFT) and autocorrelation. The FFT is used to operate the spectral analysis during PW and CW Doppler. This method can determine if the flow pattern is turbulent or normal (i.e., laminar). Autocorrelation is only used during color Doppler, but it is faster than the FFT method.

Frame Rate in B-Mode

Several factors exist that will either increase or reduce the frame rate during an ultrasound exam. If the frame rate is low, it takes longer to create an image, and a lag may be visualized in the image. Temporal resolution is the ability of the ultrasound system to track reflectors from one second to the next. When the frame rate is high, the temporal resolution is good. If the frame rate is low, the temporal resolution suffers because fewer frames are created every second. There is a direct relationship between the scanning depth and the temporal resolution. The PRF can be adjusted in B-mode via the depth button. If the depth is increased, the PRF will be lower, which means that the object being examined is deeper in the body, resulting in a decrease in the temporal resolution. If the depth is decreased, then the PRF will be higher, resulting in an increase in the temporal resolution.

Adjusting the PRF to Reduce Aliasing When Using Color Doppler

Correct optimization of color flow is always the goal when examining vessels while using color Doppler. The PRF is often referred to as the scale when Doppler is activated. Aliasing is when there is erratic color within the vessel, commonly appearing as a blue shade appearing within the red-colored section. Increasing the scale raises the Nyquist limit of the machine, eliminating the erratic color within the vessel. Aliasing can occur in color Doppler imaging and in PW imaging.

From the same site, an image showing erratic color within the vessel indicates aliasing, while an image showing a solid color filling the vessel does not. Aliasing usually occurs with stenosis; therefore, to show the lack of stenosis, sonographers should adjust the color.

Minimizing Bioeffects While Using Doppler

Sonographers should always be aware of the ALARA principle during ultrasound exams. The ALARA principle is in place to protect patients from the potential bioeffects from ultrasound. Grayscale imaging exposes the patient to the least amount of bioeffects. When color and PW Doppler are activated, the acoustic exposure risk becomes higher. The PRF would contribute to patient exposure because if the PRF is increased, more pulses are transmitted into the body, increasing the risk of acoustic exposure to the patient. If an ultrasound user notices that the Doppler signals have become really "noisy," it is because most modern systems have a built-in safety feature that will automatically reduce the output power if the PRF is too high.

Doppler Angle and Flow
Spectral Doppler
Angle Used to Maximize Doppler Shift

During routine grayscale ultrasound imaging, it has been proven that the ideal incident beam is when the transducer is placed at a 90° angle to the object being scanned. For Doppler, however, the maximum frequency shift will be obtained with an incidence angle of either 0° (i.e., the blood cells are flowing toward the transducer) or 180° (i.e., the blood cells are flowing away from the transducer). The cosine of 90° is 0, so we cannot measure any Doppler frequency when the incident beam is 90° (i.e., perpendicular) to the direction of blood flow.

$$\text{Doppler shift} = \frac{2 \times \text{velocity of blood} \times \text{frequency of transducer} \times \cos\theta}{\text{propagation speed}}$$

The cosine of 0° is 1, which correlates to the maximum Doppler shift.

Measuring Velocities When Using Spectral Doppler

For a sonographer to obtain the most accurate measurement during a vascular exam, the moving red blood cells should be located parallel to the transducer. In this case, the measurement reflects the velocity located in all parts of the ultrasound wave. A positive Doppler frequency occurs when the velocity of the returning signals from blood cells moving toward the transducer is greater than the transmitted velocity. When the blood is not moving exactly parallel to the sound beam, the velocity measurement will not be as accurate. For example, if the angle cursor is larger than the actual Doppler angle, the velocity will be too high. If the angle cursor is lower than the angle that is parallel to the vessel wall, then the velocity will be underestimated. The sample volume gate and the angle cursor are sonographer-adjustable settings on the ultrasound machine.

Crosstalk

During a spectral Doppler exam, if blood flow is visualized above and below the baseline, the sonographer should check if the flow is truly in both directions or if it is unidirectional flow. If it is unidirectional flow, this visibly bidirectional flow is an artifact called crosstalk—a specific mirror artifact that will only occur during a spectral Doppler study. Crosstalk shows an exact replica of the flow velocity on both sides of the spectral baseline. This can occur if the sonographer is attempting to obtain a velocity but the incident angle of the ultrasound wave is perpendicular to the motion of the red blood cells. Electronic mirror imaging associated with crosstalk may occur if the Doppler gain is set too high. The following image shows crosstalk during an ultrasound. Notice the identical flow above and below the baseline.

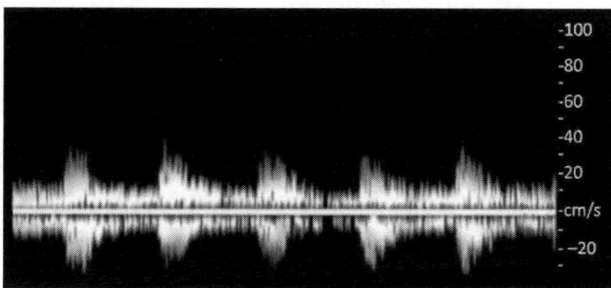

COLOR DOPPLER

If color is not displayed within a vessel after turning on color Doppler, the sonographer should immediately consider the angle of the incident beam. If the incident beam is 90° to the blood vessel being interrogated, then the color will not be visualized. According to the Doppler equation, the cosine of 90° is zero; therefore, no color can be visualized. A sonographer can improve the visualization of color Doppler by angling the color box so that the incident beam is not 90°. An ultrasound user can also decrease the scale and increase the color gain settings to increase the amount of blood visualized in the vessel.

DETERMINING THE DIRECTION OF BLOOD FLOW IN A HORIZONTAL VESSEL

Color flow in a sector-shaped image cannot be steered as it can be with a linear transducer. Only the size and location can be adjusted. If the image is sector shaped and contains a vessel that is in a horizontal direction, first, find the color map to understand what color represents blood flowing toward the transducer—the color above the black line. The color beneath the black line on the color map represents blood flowing away from the transducer. The user can then decide if the blood flow is moving from left to right or right to left by tracking the blood flow from the top color to the bottom color. This will make the direction of the blood flow more apparent.

With a linear transducer, steering the color box is essential to determine the direction of the blood flow. Another adjustment is the angle of the transducer on the skin. By rocking the transducer (or putting more weight on the heel or toe of the transducer), the sonographer can display the vessel in a more diagonal angle in order to use a better Doppler shift.

DETERMINING THE DIRECTION OF BLOOD FLOW WITH A LINEAR PROBE

The color map on the image determines which colors represent the toward flow (i.e., above the baseline) and which colors represent the away flow (i.e., beneath the baseline) in a blood vessel. When the color box is angled, it takes the shape of a parallelogram. The estimated location of the transducer within the vessel can be found by locating the top corner of the steered color box and drawing a line down. The imaginary line that does not bump into any other portion of the color box will be where the transducer is located. From the placement of the probe, determine if the color within the box is moving toward or away. The direction of blood flow is decided during tracking either to or from the position of the transducer. This will be a left-to-right or right-to-left movement.

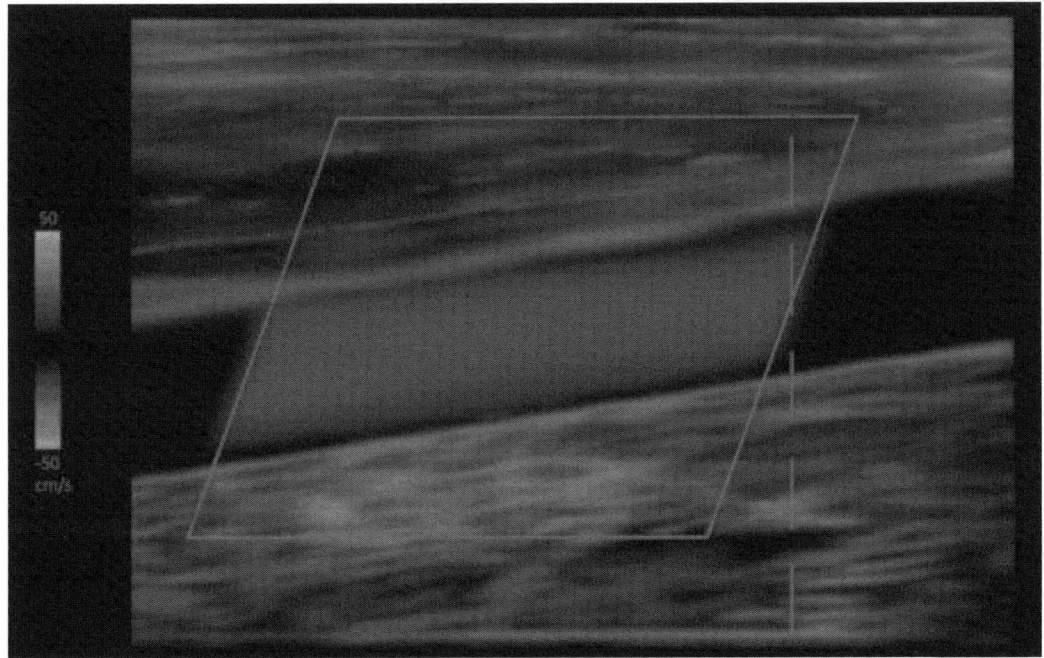

The image shows a carotid artery being scanned. The dashed line on the right of the parallelogram represents the location of the transducer. If the color shown indicates movement toward the transducer, then the blood would be moving from left to right.

Wall Filter

The **wall filter** removes Doppler shifts below a certain set frequency during spectral and color Doppler interrogations. This control will help remove the lower frequency Doppler signals that may arise from the motion that anatomical structures such as the heart or blood vessels create. Wall filters are also referred to as high-pass filters and do not affect higher Doppler shifts, such as those created from the movement of blood cells in the circulatory system. Slower moving blood will create a lower frequency Doppler shift. The system is less likely to detect blood that is moving slowly when the wall filter is set at a higher level.

Increasing the Wall Filter Setting with Color Doppler

If an ultrasound user increases the wall filter setting while using color Doppler, this will only affect the low-velocity flow in the blood vessels. In an image in which the blood flow can be seen with color Doppler in an artery and a vein and the wall filter setting is increased high enough, the arterial flow will be the only one visualized. Venous blood flow is slower than arterial flow, and by changing the wall filter (i.e., the high-pass filter) to a high setting, that removes or rejects the color Doppler from the vein. The wall filter will not affect vessels in which high-velocity flow occurs. It may, however, eliminate any ghosting artifacts that appear as color Doppler visualized on the outside lumen of a blood vessel due to the motion created by the pulsating blood vessel.

INCREASING THE WALL FILTER SETTING WITH SPECTRAL ANALYSIS

Increasing the wall filter setting during spectral analysis will only effectively remove the lower frequency Doppler shifts from slower blood flow. On a spectral Doppler waveform, lower frequency shifts are visualized near the baseline, so this is where the elimination will take place. This will not affect a sonographer's ability to measure high-velocity flows. A high wall filter level will decrease detection of slower flow. During a carotid Doppler study, if the sonographer cannot measure the velocity of the end diastolic flow, it would be beneficial to decrease the wall filter setting.

SAMPLE GATE
ADJUSTING THE COLOR BOX TO IMPROVE THE FRAME RATE DURING COLOR DOPPLER

Many controls on the ultrasound machine pertaining to the use of color Doppler and the frame rate may be adjusted during an exam. To optimize the frame rate and the temporal resolution, the user needs to be aware of the size and location of the color box. The color box will allow the velocity information to be portrayed as an overlay of color on the traditional grayscale image. As the color box size increases, the frame rate or temporal resolution decreases since more information needs to be processed. This is especially important when considering the width of the color box. More scan lines are required with a wider color box, and more time is required by the system to process the acquired data. The sonographer should limit the size of the color box to the anatomy of interest. The location is also something to consider because a deeper location may produce aliasing of the color flow because the PRF is lower.

DOPPLER PICKING UP VELOCITIES FROM AN ARTERY AND A VEIN

PW Doppler provides range resolution, which gives users a precise indication of where velocity measurements are being taken. When PW Doppler is selected on the ultrasound machine, the user will move the gate to the blood vessel to be interrogated. The size of the gate, also known as the sample volume, can be adjusted so that the user is sampling a good portion of the blood vessel. Sometimes, the sonographer will notice that blood flow from arteries and veins is being displayed. If this happens, the user can adjust the size of the gate to only obtain data from the vessel of interest. One may also have to adjust the location because an unsteady hand can move off of the artery or vein. Modern systems will have a triplex function that allows the user to display grayscale, color Doppler, and spectral Doppler at the same time. If the transducer is picking up flow from two different vessels, the user can update the triplex image and move the sample volume into the vessel under investigation.

COLOR DOPPLER MAP

Color maps are an important diagnostic tool when using color Doppler during an ultrasound exam. The operator must pay close attention to the colors that are represented in the map because they portray information about the direction of flow as well as the velocity. The color map will be visualized along the side of the image once the color Doppler is turned on. For example, if red is displayed at the top of the color map and blue is at the bottom, then there will be a black line between the two colors that represents an area in which a Doppler shift is not present. The colors in the upper half of the color map represent blood that is moving toward the transducer. The colors beneath the black line represent blood flow that is moving away from the probe.

If a color map contains multiple colors, the user can discern the velocities of the flow moving toward the transducer. The colors that are closer to the top show blood flow that is traveling at a higher velocity than those near the black line in the middle of the map.

Variance Mode Map

A variance mode map gives the sonographer information not only about the direction and velocity of red blood cells in the sample but also about the flow pattern of the blood. Similar to velocity mode maps, variance mode maps have a black line that represents an area where no Doppler shift occurs. Above this black line is flow moving toward the probe, and below the black line is flow moving away from the probe. However, the boxes above and below the black line contain different colors on each side. Recall that normal flow in a vessel is considered laminar flow, which is represented by flow on the left of the color map. Turbulent flow is the opposite of laminar flow and is found on the right side of the color map. An example of turbulent flow may be the result of blood flow moving through a stenotic vessel.

The gradient of color changes correlates to the colors within the vessel. A higher speed within the vessel will be a slightly different shade from a slower speed within the vessel.

Types of Doppler

Continuous Wave (CW)

A method of Doppler interrogation that uses two crystals—one to transmit and the other to receive the pulse—is known as continuous-wave (CW) Doppler. This method is used to gain accurate velocities of rapid blood flow. It can also be used to eliminate aliasing. Because aliasing never occurs with CW Doppler, a sonographer can more confidently and accurately measure peak velocity blood flow. Dedicated CW transducers do not generate images, but they are very sensitive and can pick up small Doppler shifts, so they are used when trying to find flow in small vessels in the extremities.

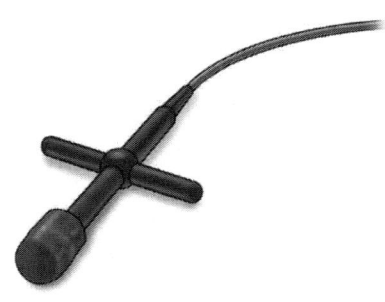

CW Transducer Sensitivity

Dedicated CW transducers are more sensitive to signals that are weaker within the body because these probes do not contain backing (i.e., damping) material. Backing material inhibits the amount of ringing of the crystals during the transmitting and receiving phases, which makes them less receptive to receiving returning signals that tend to be smaller. If these tiny signals are not recognized by the transducer, then the ultrasound system cannot convert them into electrical signals to be visualized on the screen. Dedicated CW probes are great for detecting tiny Doppler shifts, such as blood flow in the foot. Matching layers are present in dedicated CW probes to more readily allow for the propagation of sound in and out of the body.

Overcoming Aliasing with CW Doppler

Aliasing is an error in imaging that occurs when using PW Doppler if the waveform winds around the top or bottom of the display. Aliasing takes place when the Doppler shift is greater than the Nyquist limit, which is half of the PRF. Aliasing only occurs with PW Doppler (which includes both color and PW spectral Doppler). Using CW Doppler is one of methods used to overcome aliasing. There is no listening time with these transducers; therefore, there is no limit on the frequency shift (i.e., there is no Nyquist limit).

Measuring Peak Blood Flow Velocity

PW Doppler measures blood flow velocities within various blood vessels. The ultrasound user has the option to select where the gate should be placed within a vessel to take a velocity measurement and know the exact location of this reading; however, sometimes, the velocity within the blood vessel is too high and the operator is unable to obtain an accurate peak velocity measurement. Switching to CW Doppler will allow for more accurate measurements of the high velocities because there is no maximum velocity with this method. While using PW Doppler, if the user cannot eliminate aliasing after changing the scale or depth of the target and switching to a lower frequency probe, CW Doppler can be used instead.

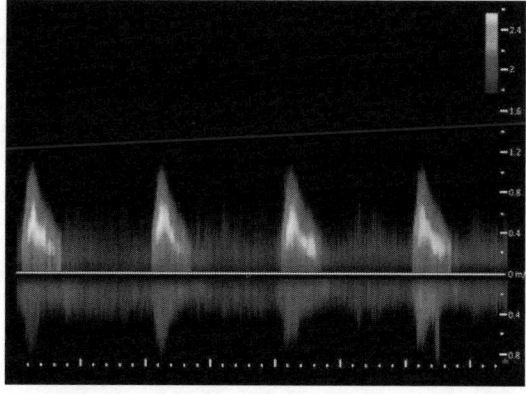

The image shows a CW Doppler reading. Note the lack of image, consistent with CW transducers. Just the waveform is seen, leading to an increase in sensitivity of the readings.

Disadvantages of CW Doppler

Range resolution is the capability of determining the precise location at which an ultrasound machine obtained a velocity measurement in the body. This is also referred to as range specificity. To know exactly where the measurement is taken, the operator will use a gate (i.e., a sample volume) that will appear on the grayscale and color Doppler image. Range resolution is also offered by color Doppler as a determination of the location of blood flow. CW Doppler does not, however, offer range resolution: the spectral analysis obtained with this technique suffers from range ambiguity artifact, which is when the sample is an unknown depth due to the lack of image. Although very high velocities can accurately be measured with CW Doppler, the signals that are received arise from the entire line that was positioned on the screen.

Pulsed Wave (PW)

When performing a PW Doppler exam, the sonographer can determine exactly where a velocity measurement should be taken within a vessel. Once the sonographer has the grayscale image optimized, color Doppler can be activated to better visualize the blood vessels. Then, the user can bring up the cursor for PW Doppler, and a line that is intersected by two dashes close together will be visualized. This is the gate (i.e., the sample volume), which can be moved with the trackball until it is exactly where the user wants to perform a spectral analysis. The size of the gate can be changed so that it is only within the vessel that is being examined. For example, when sampling the carotid artery but the spectral display is also showing venous flow, the user will reduce the size of the gate and reposition it so that only the artery is being interrogated.

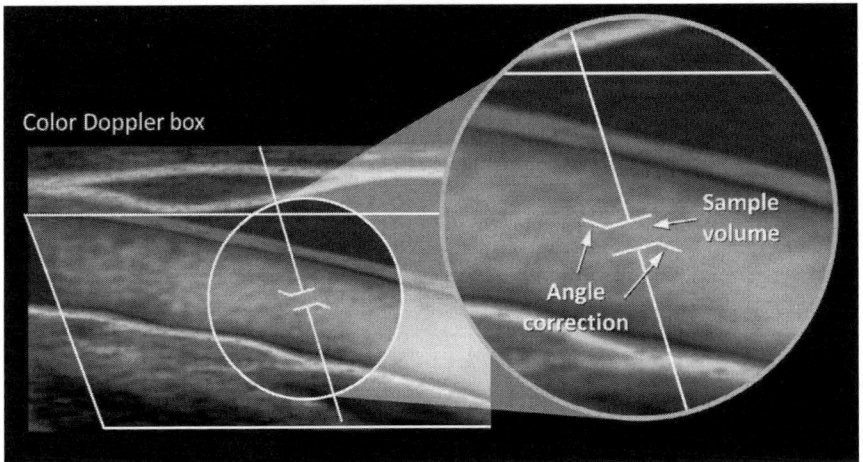

This image shows the sample volume and angle correction within the vessel. The angle correction feature is shown by the little wings that come out from the sample volume. It is meant to be adjusted parallel to the vessel to obtain an accurate velocity reading.

Transducer Type for PW Doppler

PW Doppler only requires one active element. This piezoelectric lead zirconate titanate (PZT) crystal can transmit the pulse into the body as well as listen for the returning signals. Only one PZT crystal is necessary because the sonographer places the sample volume (i.e., the gate) in exactly the position at which a sample velocity is necessary. Once the probe transmits a pulse into the body, it listens for it to return to the transducer. This is known as the time of flight (i.e., the go-return time). Transducers that allow PW Doppler are also able to create a grayscale image: this is referred to as duplex/triplex imaging.

Adjusting the PRF to Improve PW Doppler Visualization

The PRF is also referred to as the scale while PW Doppler is being used. This can be adjusted to improve PW Doppler visualization. For example, if the vessel being interrogated displays blood flow that is moving slowly and the color is not optimized after turning on color Doppler, the sonographer would decrease the PRF so that the ultrasound system is more receptive in picking up slower blood flow signals. The venous portion of the circulatory system is often where slow blood flow will be seen. If this step alone does not improve color Doppler visualization of the vessel, then the sonographer may need to increase the color gain. If the operator chooses to increase the PRF scale, he or she would notice a decreased sensitivity to slow flow states; however, when interrogating a vessel with higher velocity flow, the PRF should be set higher to raise the Nyquist limit and prevent or eliminate aliasing.

Advantages of a Superficial Sample Volume

The PRF is the number of pulses that an ultrasound machine can send into the body per second. During PW Doppler applications, the system is required to send out multiple pulses each second to get the best possible velocity measurements, and PRF is the sampling rate that is offered by the machine. If the sample volume is superficial (i.e., shallow), the velocity can be sampled many times per second, so the velocity readings are considered quite precise. Samples that arise from structures that are not very deep in the body will create a high PRF and a high Nyquist limit. Aliasing is less likely to occur at more superficial depths than when trying to image structures located deeper in the body. If the reflectors are deeper, it requires a lower PRF, which also lowers the Nyquist limit. Recall that the Nyquist limit is referred to as the aliasing frequency.

Disadvantage of PW Doppler

One major disadvantage of PW Doppler is its inability to accurately measure high-velocity blood flow. When incorrectly portrayed, high-velocity flow will appear to wrap around the spectral window and seem as if it is moving in the wrong direction. This phenomenon is known as aliasing and is a misrepresentation that is frequently seen with PW Doppler. While using PW Doppler, the sonographer should be aware of steps to take to eliminate aliasing. These include adjusting the scale to a reasonable velocity, adjusting the baseline, selecting a lower frequency, and finding a window that will be in a shallower location.

INTERMITTENT SAMPLING AND ALIASING ARTIFACTS

Aliasing is common during PW Doppler exams due to intermittent sampling, which occurs if the Doppler frequency is not evaluated correctly. When the Doppler frequency is larger than the Nyquist limit, aliasing will take place. Aliasing can also arise when color Doppler is being used, so sonographers should be able to identify the artifact if it is present.

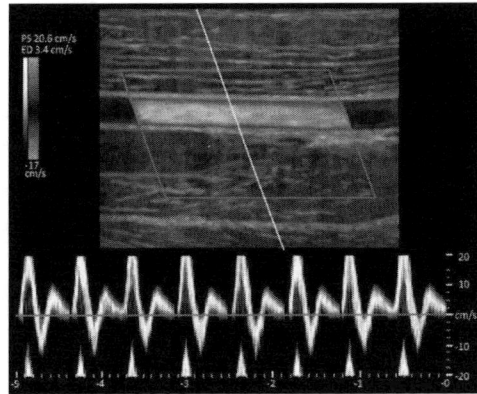

Notice how the waveform is cut off on the top of the spectral image and wraps around on the bottom of the image. The wrapping around of the waveform is spectral aliasing, not to be confused with color aliasing.

TRANSDUCER SELECTION AND ALIASING ARTIFACTS

Aliasing will be eliminated when a lower frequency transducer is used because it will have smaller Doppler shifts. Higher frequency probes are more prone to aliasing artifacts. Because the Doppler shift is calculated using the frequency of the transducer, this in turn will have a direct relationship. Recall that aliasing is when the spectral waveform tends to wind around the spectral window, but the height of the spectrum will be less when a lower frequency transducer is used for an exam. The same transducer can be used for duplex imaging, so the grayscale image may suffer because of the lower frequency. Modern probes allow for multiple frequencies, so the ultrasound user can easily toggle between higher and lower frequencies during an exam with the same transducer.

NYQUIST LIMIT WITH PW DOPPLER

The Nyquist limit can be calculated by dividing the PRF by 2. Aliasing will be apparent if the Doppler frequency is higher than the Nyquist limit. Therefore, to prevent aliasing, the sonographer will raise the Nyquist limit. This can be done by raising the PRF scale: if the PRF is increased, so is the Nyquist limit. One may also raise the Nyquist limit by finding a new, more shallow sonographic window. The PRF is determined by the depth of the reflector. If the reflector is deeper in the body, the PRF will be low, as will the Nyquist limit. This decreased value makes the ultrasound system more susceptible to aliasing.

$$\text{Nyquist limit (Hz)} = \frac{\text{PRF (Hz)}}{2}$$

Color Doppler

Packet Size

The packet size is the number of pulses transmitted in a color scan line in color Doppler. Packets are used to get precise measurements of the velocities of moving blood cells. The packet size may also be called the ensemble length, or shots per line. A sonographer should be aware of the advantages and disadvantages of changing the packet size during color Doppler interrogation, especially regarding the temporal resolution and obtaining accurate measurements.

Adjusting the Packet Size

The velocity of blood flow can be more true to form if the packet size is increased, but the frame rate may suffer as a result. Color Doppler requires every scan line to be pulsed more than once. The packet size (i.e., the ensemble length, or shots per line) represents these numerous pulses sent out for each scan line. The packet size can be raised when trying to image smaller vessels that are within the venous system because the ultrasound machine will be able to detect low-flow states more readily.

Packet size can be adjusted through the settings of the ultrasound machine. It is adjusted by changing the PRF, the sample volume size, and the number of pulses being sent. Increasing the PRF and the sample volume size and therefore increasing the number of pulses being sent will increase the packet size. While there is not a specific knob to make this modification, it is an accumulation of adjustments that can be made to accommodate the Doppler image.

Increasing the Frame Rate

A sonographer should decrease the packet size when interrogating organs with color Doppler in order to increase the frame rate. Multiple packets are used during color Doppler scans to increase the sensitivity to low flow and to get a more precise measurement of the velocities; however, there are disadvantages associated with an increased packet size, including a decrease in the temporal resolution. More pulses being sent out at the same time tends to reduce the frame rate and requires more time for data acquisition.

Scale

A sonographer can successfully remove aliasing artifacts when using color Doppler by changing the velocity scale. If the scale is set too low but the velocities that are detected are high-flow vessels, then aliasing may occur. The most efficient way to eliminate aliasing is by increasing the velocity scale. This step may, however, decrease the sensitivity of the color flow to vessels in which low-flow velocities are found. Another way to remove aliasing from an image on color Doppler is to switch to a lower frequency transducer, which will enable better penetration and be less likely to alias.

Gain

Color Doppler with an Anemic Patient

If a patient is anemic, he or she has a lower than normal amount of red blood cells circulating in the blood. Some patients may be anemic because they do not have enough hemoglobin in their blood. Hemoglobin is a protein that contains iron, which transports oxygen from the lungs to all of the body's cells. A patient with anemia will still have enough red blood cells in the circulatory system to be able to successfully undergo a color Doppler exam. For diagnostic ultrasound imaging, the main reflectors that provide information pertaining to Doppler frequencies are the red blood cells. Because the blood is constantly being transported throughout the heart and blood vessels, even a patient that is anemic will have enough red blood cells for a successful Doppler exam.

Adjusting Color Doppler Gain

If a sonographer cannot visualize color during a carotid duplex exam, the first thing that can be done is to determine the angle of the color box with the direction of blood flow. It is important for sonographers to remember that if the color box is perpendicular (i.e., at a 90° angle) to a vessel, color will never be visualized. Modern systems allow color boxes to be steered with linear transducers, which will prevent the beam from being perpendicular to the vessel. Next, the user can increase the color gain. This demonstrates the amplification of signals within blood vessels, but it will not show blood flow if it is not actually present. The velocity scale is also important to adjust if blood flow is not well demonstrated or if aliasing occurs.

Optimal Setting for Color Doppler Gain

If a sonographer visualizes multiple speckled colors throughout the color box after turning on color Doppler, the first step that he or she can take to correct this noise is to turn the color gain down. Color gain that is set correctly is adjusted so that the amplitude is set at the highest level without displaying color speckles. Aliasing, color Doppler gain that is set too high, and turbulent flow all have different appearances, so ultrasound users should be able to discern what is taking place. Some are artifacts and can be corrected with the adjustment of parameters on the ultrasound machine.

Aliasing with Color Doppler

Color Doppler uses grayscale imaging to locate anatomical structures, and, when activated, a color box will be layered on top of the B-mode image. This information includes data about the mean velocity of blood moving through various structures instead of peak velocity as measured by PW and CW Doppler. Color Doppler does provide information regarding the direction of blood flow, and it is prone to aliasing. Ultrasound users should be able to tell the difference between color Doppler that is aliasing and flow that is moving in the reverse direction. The operator must pay close attention to the color map displayed on the screen. Just as PW Doppler that is aliasing tends to wrap around the spectral window, color Doppler that is aliasing winds around the top of the color box around to the bottom.

POWER DOPPLER IMAGING (PDI)

Power Doppler imaging (also called energy mode or color angiography) is a form of color Doppler that does not display the speed of blood flow or any directional information. Rather, it determines that a Doppler shift has taken place and shows the amplitude of the moving blood. If there are more red blood cells in one area, the signals will be brighter. Vessels represented with PDI will all be identical colors on the display. Advantages of PDI include the fact that aliasing does not occur because the speed and direction of blood flow are not applicable. PDI picks up blood flow in smaller vessels and it picks up slow blood flow because of its increased sensitivity. There is an increase in sensitivity because PDI is not altered by the Doppler angle. The disadvantages of PDI are due to the increased sensitivity: flash artifact may be visualized when the patient moves or breathes. PDI does not evaluate the direction or velocity of the blood flow. When compared to color Doppler, the temporal resolution is greatly reduced.

FLASH ARTIFACT

A disadvantage of PDI is that the study may suffer because of flash artifact. Flash artifact does not occur because of the motion of the red blood cells; rather, it is a burst of color visualized when there is motion taking place outside of the blood vessels. Often, this motion is caused by patient movement. Examples of patient motion include voluntary movement, like the patient moving on the exam table, but it may also be involuntary motion, such as movement of the heart or lungs during respiration. Flash artifact may also appear because of motion caused by the transducer as the sonographer is moving it on the patient or even motion caused from the pressure that the transducer places on soft-tissue structures. Flash artifact may appear as a randomized burst of color, occurring outside of the vessels.

SPECTRAL DOPPLER
SPECTRAL ANALYSIS

Spectral analysis provides information pertaining to the individual velocities of blood cells that are contained within a specific sample. Spectral analysis is a tool that simplifies the many Doppler shifts that are produced when blood travels through the body. Blood does not travel in a uniform fashion, and, because of this, spectral analysis is necessary to provide data that can offer diagnostic information to correctly diagnose patients that suffer from vascular disease. Sonographers realize that even within the same blood vessel that is free of any pathology, the blood moves at different speeds. When pathology is present or the vessels change shapes and sizes, the flow patterns can change dramatically. Spectral analysis allows users to visually sort out all of this information along with measuring various velocities.

SPECTRAL BROADENING

A spectral Doppler waveform represents all of the many velocities found in a sample of a blood vessel. Spectral Doppler allows sonographers to see, hear, and measure various blood flow velocities. Two types of flow can be ascertained in the sample: (1) normal or laminar flow, in which the spectral window is clear and the red blood cells are traveling at almost the same velocities, and (2) turbulent flow, which shows disorganized flow because the blood is traveling at different speeds and in various directions. Instead of a clear spectral window as seen in laminar flow, spectral broadening results in the window appearing to be filled in. Spectral broadening is typical when turbulent (i.e., high-velocity) blood flow is sampled. This turbulence comprises many areas of flow reversal and various velocities, and flow may be seen beneath the baseline. Spectral broadening is a display of a broad range of Doppler shifts that are apparent within the sample of blood flow taken in a vessel. This may happen due to a stenosis or a tortuous vessel.

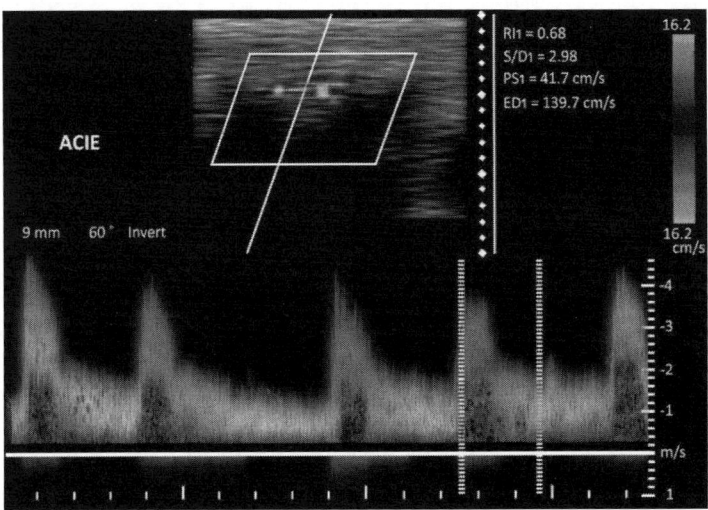

The image shows atherosclerotic disease in the common carotid arteries. If you look at the waveform below the image, you can see spectral broadening, identified by the filling of the waveform to the baseline.

CORRECTING AN ALIASING ARTIFACT

Spectral Doppler waveforms can provide clinicians with much insight pertaining to blood flowing throughout the body. Blood does not necessarily travel in the same speed or direction, even within the same blood vessel. Spectral analysis identifies every velocity obtained within the signal that is reflected. However, when there are aliasing errors in the spectral waveform, the interpreting physician may mistake that data as true information. This could lead to a misdiagnosis. In such cases, the sonographer may attempt to reduce aliasing by reducing the transducer's Doppler frequency. The PRF scale could also be increased to raise the Nyquist limit, and the baseline could be moved down. If that does not work, the user could increase the angle of incidence or switch to CW Doppler.

COMBINING PW AND COLOR DOPPLER

An advantage of PW Doppler is that the user knows exactly where the blood flow velocity is being sampled because of the gate. Color Doppler allows information pertaining to the velocities to be superimposed on a grayscale image. Color Doppler also allows users to determine in which direction the blood is traveling. Using PW Doppler and color Doppler allows the sonographer to experience the benefits of both methods. Using both methods correlates the color Doppler blood flow with specific quantities in the pulsed wave, helping to identify high-velocity flow at specific speeds.

GAIN

PW Doppler provides important information that can be used to diagnose many disorders in patients. Correct Doppler settings are crucial, and sonographers must have a strong understanding of not only human anatomy but also of ultrasound physics. If the machine is not set properly, an artifact can occur that may limit the amount of diagnostic information present. If a sonographer turns on the PW Doppler, but the spectral display can barely be visualized, then the next step will be to turn up the PW Doppler's gain. If the gain is turned up too high, then noise may appear in the spectral display. One can increase the gain by turning it up until noise appears. At this point, the gain may be slowly reduced until the noise disappears.

ULTRASOUND NOISE

A sonographer should be aware of various spectral Doppler artifacts so that the results are not misconstrued. The parameters on the ultrasound machine should be understood and set correctly so that information is not lost or added to the image. Noise is one such artifact that can degrade the quality of the spectral waveform. Noise can typically be identified easily by the user and can be alleviated by reducing the amount of the PW Doppler gain. Noise may appear like spectral broadening, which could cause the interpreting physician to incorrectly diagnose it as turbulent flow. The user should turn down the gain so that the spectral window is clear but the systolic and diastolic components can easily be visualized along with forward flow patterns.

This is like ghosting on color Doppler. Ultrasound noise artifact can be eliminated by lowering the PW gain or by increasing the wall filter.

TISSUE DOPPLER IMAGING (TDI)

Tissue Doppler imaging (TDI) is used in several cardiac ultrasound applications. This is a technique that may be underused and could be used as a screening method for patients with heart dysfunction. An advantage of TDI is the sensitivity that it grants sonographers in routine cardiac imaging, which is especially useful when considering therapeutic intervention. TDI is offered by most ultrasound vendors on dedicated cardiac systems. TDI allows for the collection of quantitative data of myocardial function during stress and at rest. TDI has great potential in the diagnosis of diastolic left ventricular heart defects. It can be used to interrogate systolic and diastolic function, heart failure, cardiomyopathy, diseases of the heart valves, and determining if patients would be candidates for a defibrillator or pacemaker.

ELASTOGRAPHY IMAGING

Elastography provides quick and painless measurements of the stiffness of an organ or tissue being interrogated. Stiffness data from elastography are combined with ultrasound data to create a diagnosis. B-mode and color Doppler can also be used in conjunction with the elastogram to provide even more information for the clinician. Shear-wave elastography distorts the tissue by using the pressure that propagates from the sound wave instead of requiring the sonographer to apply external pressure. Transient elastography of the liver, for example, would require a perpendicular approach from the intercostal region. Once a window is found away from large vessels, the probe button is activated to begin obtaining data. Typically, it is believed that benign structures tend to be softer than their stiffer, malignant counterparts. This dynamic technique continues to be evaluated to determine its diagnostic capability. Elastography offers additional information for breast lesions, liver fibrosis, and musculoskeletal imaging.

Doppler Measurements

RED BLOOD CELLS

Blood is composed of many components, including red blood cells (i.e., erythrocytes), white blood cells (i.e., leukocytes), platelets (i.e., thrombocytes), and plasma. Roughly 45% of the blood that travels throughout the circulatory system (i.e., the heart, arteries, capillaries, and veins) comprises red blood cells. Red blood cells supply oxygen to all of the cells in the body, and they are the most numerous type of cell in whole blood. The life span of red blood cells is about 120 days, but they are constantly being replenished by new red blood cells. Because red blood cells are traveling in the heart and blood vessels, they create the reflections that are seen by the human eye when color Doppler is turned on (sometimes the blood flow can be seen, especially in low-flow states, without color Doppler).

DOPPLER SHIFT

In general, a Doppler shift is produced when an ultrasound wave collides with a red blood cell that is in motion. When the red blood cells are moving in the direction of the transducer, the result is a reflected frequency that is greater than the frequency of the transmitted signal. This demonstrates a positive Doppler shift (aka the Doppler frequency). If the red blood cells are moving in the opposite direction of the transducer, a negative Doppler shift would take place. The amount of Doppler shift that occurs is directly proportional to the frequency of the transducer. Therefore, if an exam is repeated with a transducer that has a frequency that is twice as high as what was used in the first exam, the Doppler shift will be doubled.

When using ultrasound for diagnostic purposes, the frequency of the transducers used during a Doppler exam range from approximately 2–10 MHz. The formula to calculate Doppler shift is as follows:

$$\text{Doppler shift} = \text{reflected frequency} - \text{transmitted frequency}$$

The Doppler shift is directly related to the velocity of blood within the circulatory system. The velocity includes the speed (i.e., the magnitude) and direction of blood flow. Slower velocities will cause a lower Doppler frequency. A higher velocity will create a greater Doppler shift. Blood flow velocities are reported in units of meters per second (m/s).

LAMINAR FLOW

Laminar flow is exhibited in normal anatomical structures. If a clinician listens to the blood moving through a vessel with laminar flow, it will not be heard. This flow is layered and smooth, and it travels parallel along the length of the vessel. There are two configurations regarding laminar flow. The first is plug flow, which will have the same velocity in all layers. The second is parabolic flow, which tends to have velocities that are higher in the middle of the vessel and lower along the vessel walls. A parabolic flow pattern creates a shape like a bullet. A blood vessel that contains laminar flow will produce a Reynolds number of less than 1,500. The Reynolds number is a way to forecast if the flow will be laminar or turbulent. Turbulent flow will have a Reynolds number that is greater than 2,000.

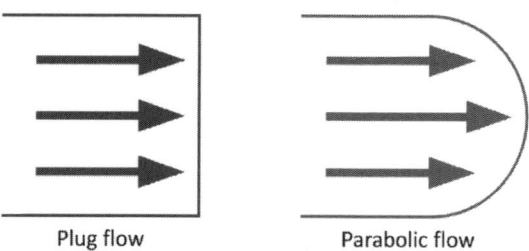

The image depicts the two different laminar flow types. The structure on the left shows plug flow, in which all the layers travel at the same velocity. The image on the right shows parabolic flow, in which the velocity is the highest in the center, gradually decreasing to the slowest speed at the vessel's walls.

DIFFERENTIATING BLOOD FLOW TYPES

Three types of blood flow seen in the circulatory systems of humans are phasic, pulsatile, and steady. Phasic flow is the typical flow pattern seen in veins, which can vary due to respiration. Steady flow is when the blood is moving at a constant velocity, and it occurs in venous circulation when respiration is paused. Pulsatile flow occurs when the movement of blood is dependent on cardiac contraction. Pulsatile flow is seen more commonly in arterial blood flow.

An example of pulsatile flow is seen with echocardiography, in which the heart is contracting. Phasic flow is seen in veins. Steady (nonphasic) flow can be seen when the patient holds their breath during a pulse Doppler of the portal vein in an abdominal study.

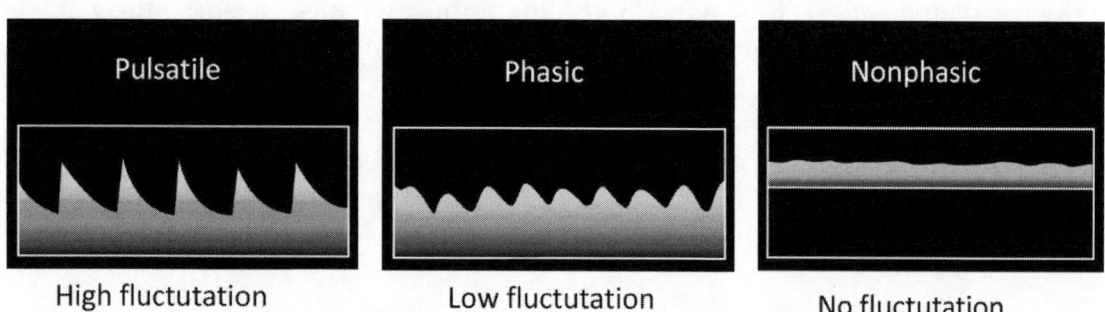

POSTSTENOTIC TURBULENCE

Patent refers to a structure that is open, or clear. If a vessel is not patent, there may be a blockage, stenosis, or clot. If a sonographer visualizes a stenosis on routine grayscale imaging, a narrowing of the blood vessel lumen (i.e., the opening) is present. If the user adds color Doppler, the direction of flow may vary because the blood is attempting to enter and exit the stenotic region of the blood vessel. When PW Doppler is used, the sonographer may expect to obtain higher flow velocities within the stenosis, but an even greater measurement distal to the stenosis. This is known as poststenotic turbulence, which is located after the blood vessel has been narrowed. Eddy currents will likely be visualized because the blood is no longer moving as smoothly as it was before the stenosis. If a clinician listens to the blood flow in this region, a bruit may be revealed.

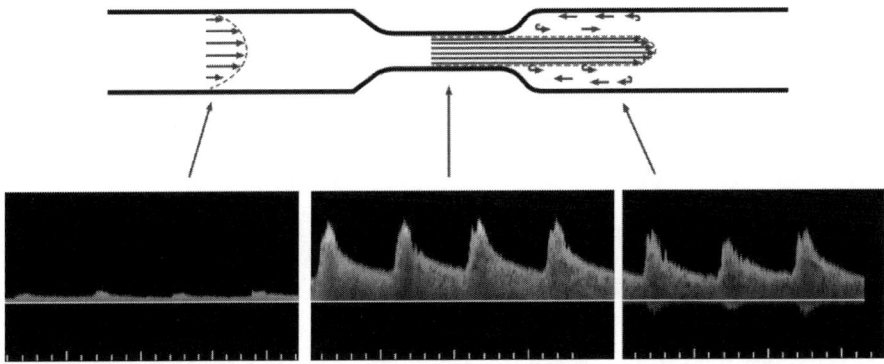

If you look at this vessel, before the stenosis (the narrowing in the middle of the vessel), there is normal parabolic flow on the left. On the right of the image, look at the turbulent, chaotic flow that occurs after stenosis. If you correlate it with PW Doppler, you will see the normal flow on the left, the high-velocity flow in the middle with stenosis, and the chaotic flow with spectral broadening on the right.

REYNOLDS NUMBER

The Reynolds number is a value that predicts the onset of turbulent flow. The Reynolds number is a unitless value that is calculated with the following equation:

$$\text{Reynolds number} = \frac{\text{average flow speed} \times \text{vessel diameter} \times \text{density}}{\text{viscosity}}$$

If the calculated value is less than 1,500, laminar flow will be present. If the value is more than 2,000, it is predicted that a turbulent flow will be visualized. Disturbed flow will fall between the 1,500 and 2,000 range. From the above equation, if there is an increased speed of flow, there will be a higher Reynolds number. If the diameter of the vessel is larger, then the Reynolds number will also be greater. Density has the same effect on the Reynolds number. The Reynolds number has an indirect relationship with the viscosity of the blood.

Artifacts

SPECTRAL DOPPLER

PRF AND SCALE

Many parameters can be controlled by the sonographer to prevent aliasing during an exam. One of these is to change the PRF scale. Remember that aliasing occurs if the measured frequency shift is greater than the Nyquist limit. The Nyquist limit is equal to half of the PRF. If the PRF is adjusted higher, the Nyquist limit will also be higher. However, with extremely high velocity blood flow, even if the PRF is maximized, aliasing may still occur. If this occurs, the sonographer could switch to CW Doppler because aliasing does not take place when it is used. Users should be aware that when maximizing the PRF scale, the system may not recognize vessels with slower blood flow.

ADJUSTING THE BASELINE

During a spectral display, the system can document flow that is moving in opposite directions. Flow that is visualized above the baseline demonstrates flow that is moving toward the transducer. Flow below the baseline signifies blood flowing away from the transducer. If the user notices that the flow is wrapping around the baseline, this is an aliasing artifact. Sonographers can take many steps to eliminate aliasing. One such corrective measure that can be done is to adjust the baseline. If the flow is above the baseline but aliasing occurs, the user can move the baseline lower so that the entire waveform is going in one direction. This allows for extremely high velocity flow to be shown moving in the correct direction, and it still allows for an accurate measurement.

COLOR DOPPLER

DIFFERENTIATE BETWEEN FLOW REVERSAL AND ALIASING WITH COLOR DOPPLER

It is important for sonographers to realize that aliasing can occur not only with spectral Doppler analysis, but also with color Doppler. The user must be able to discern between aliasing and the reversal of flow (i.e., bidirectional flow). To determine if aliasing is present, the user must pay close attention to the color map located on the side of the image. If the colors on the map tend to wrap from the top around the outside and to the bottom of the map, then users may assume that aliasing is present. If the colors on the middle of the color map communicate with each other, then bidirectional flow is present. The most effective step that an ultrasound user can take to remove an aliasing artifact from a color Doppler exam is to increase the level of the velocity scale.

TURBULENT FLOW AND WALL FILTERS

If a sonographer notices turbulent flow within an artery, increasing the wall filter will not remove the turbulent appearance of this flow. Wall filters are useful when trying to eliminate ghosting artifacts that are sometimes visualized during color Doppler exams. If ghosting is visualized, it will appear as color that is seen outside of the vessel. If a wall filter is activated, then the smaller Doppler shifts are excluded. Sonographers would never want turbulent flow to disappear from an image, if it is indeed present while applying a wall filter. Turbulence can add important diagnostic information when a diseased vessel is present. The presence of a wall filter will modify the flow that is seen in veins, however. For example, if a sonographer is imaging a carotid artery and he or she can see blood flow in the adjacent jugular vein but applies a wall filter, the flow in the vessel will be removed, but even high-velocity flow will be seen in the carotid artery.

Clinical Safety and Quality Assurance

Clinical Safety

UNIVERSAL INFECTION CONTROL PROTOCOLS

An ultrasound technologist plays a crucial role in applying universal infection control protocols—not only to protect their patients, but also to protect themselves. The following are key practices in implementing these protocols:

Hand hygiene: It is important to perform thorough hand hygiene practices before and after each patient interaction. Hands should be washed with soap and water for at least 20 seconds. The use of hand sanitizers is also permissible when soap is not readily available. Proper hand hygiene is a powerful measure to prevent the spread of infection.

Personal protective equipment (PPE): PPE is used frequently in clinical interactions to protect against potential infections. This includes gowns, gloves, masks, and eye protection. Understanding the appropriate type of PPE for each situation is essential to create a barrier against potential contaminants. For example, gloves should always be used during ultrasound examinations and should be discarded immediately after.

Equipment disinfection: Ultrasound equipment is a key tool in patient care and therefore requires regular cleaning and disinfection. Different surfaces require different cleaning procedures and disinfectants. For instance, an ultrasound transducer may require the use of a different type of disinfectant wipe.

Patient preparation: Proper patient preparation is vital. Ensure the proper use of clean linens, drapes, and sterile gel for all patient interactions. By ensuring a sterile environment during ultrasound examinations, the risk of infection is significantly reduced.

Waste disposal: Responsible waste disposal is also an important part of controlling infections. Always discard used PPE and other single-use items according to facility-specific protocols.

Respiratory hygiene and cough etiquette: Respiratory hygiene involves the use of common practices to minimize the transmission of respiratory infections. It involves behaviors such as covering the mouth or nose with a tissue or elbow when sneezing or coughing. Used tissues should always be disposed of appropriately in a lined trash can. Wearing a mask can also help prevent the transmission of respiratory droplets.

DISINFECTION OF ENDOCAVITY PROBES

Sonographers can prevent nosocomial (hospital-acquired) infections by using probe covers on the endocavity transducer. Once the protective covering is applied, the user should look for any tears or cracks. Upon removal from the body, the probe cover is removed, excess gel is wiped off, and the transducer is disinfected with a germicide. This process is considered to be high-level disinfection. CIDEX OPA is a common disinfectant agent used in ultrasound labs for endocavity transducers (see the solution information regarding the amount of time necessary for disinfecting). Regardless of the type of transducer that is used, it is important to properly disinfect it between patients. For those transducers that are not inserted into a patient, low-level disinfection will suffice. The ultrasound manufacturer will recommend certain cleaning solutions to prevent damage to the transducer.

CDC GUIDELINES

Maintaining patient safety during ultrasound procedures is crucial. This means adhering to Centers for Disease Control and Prevention (CDC) guidelines and ensuring the highest standards of preventing and controlling infections.

According to the CDC, vaginal and endocavity probes without covers are considered **semicritical** due to their direct contact with mucous membranes. It is highly advised to use a new condom or probe cover for each patient along with high-level disinfection. **High-level disinfection** for ultrasound probes refers to a rigorous process of disinfecting the probe to eliminate bacteria, viruses, and fungi. This is necessary for any probe that comes into direct contact with mucous membranes or sterile body sites during ultrasound procedures. Sonographers should also be aware that probe covers and condoms can fail; therefore, high-level disinfection is still necessary despite using a cover. High-level disinfection in healthcare facilities can involve chemical disinfectants or even automated probe disinfection systems. Ultrasound probes that are used during surgical procedures should also be covered with a sterile sheath to prevent contamination. If a transducer cover is damaged during any procedure, it should be immediately discarded and replaced with a new cover. To prevent infection transmission, routine disinfection between each examination is emphasized.

The CDC advises the use of **single-use sterile ultrasound gel packets** during transcutaneous procedures, as opposed to nonsterile ultrasound gel bottles. This includes procedures such as amniocentesis and paracentesis. If multiuse gel bottles must be used, it is advised to not allow the bottle tip to come into contact with the patient, probe, or any equipment. This is to prevent patient cross-contamination and also the contamination of the ultrasound gel. Refilling and heating of gel bottles is also discouraged since it can lead to cross-contamination, growth of microorganisms, and transmission of pathogens. It is also recommended to implement comprehensive cleaning/disinfection protocols for ultrasound devices. This ensures the prevention of infections and maintaining a hygienic environment in healthcare.

By incorporating these guidelines into routine practices, sonographers can contribute to a safer ultrasound process, prioritizing the well-being of themselves and their patients and upholding high standards of care.

Instrument Checks

TRANSDUCER INTEGRITY

The ultrasound transducer is a critical component of the daily work of a sonographer, and it is important to ensure its accuracy and reliability for diagnostic imaging. Assessing transducer integrity should include visual inspection and functional testing.

- **Visual inspection**—Examine the cables, connectors, and housing for noticeable signs of physical damage, cracks, or discoloration. Assess the front surface of the transducer for scratches and cracks. Make sure that the transducer cables and connectors are secure and have no signs of kinks, fraying, or looseness.
- **Functional testing**—Evaluate image resolution, assess penetration, and identify possible artifacts with a tissue-equivalent phantom.

Document and address any noted issues promptly.

USING A PHASED-ARRAY TRANSDUCER WITH A DEFECTIVE CRYSTAL

If a sonographer is using a convex phased-array transducer, the image will appear as a sector shape that is blunted at the top. If that probe has a defective element, the user will see a vertical band of dropout directly under the affected crystal. A convex (curvilinear) probe contains numerous (120–250) pieces of active elements arranged beside each other in a curved line. The PZT elements are activated in groups, sending out beams that are straight ahead, but the arced shape creates beams that are sent out in various directions. Linear sequential arrays are always parallel to each other because of the flat shape of the probe. If a sonographer is using an annular phased-array transducer with one damaged ring, there will be a horizontal band of dropout across the ultrasound image.

USING A MECHANICAL TRANSDUCER WITH A DEFECTIVE CRYSTAL

If a sonographer is using a mechanical transducer, it should be known that there is only one active element used to create an image. The shape of an image formed by a mechanical transducer is a sector, or fan-shaped, image. The beam is steered mechanically and has fixed beam focusing. Because this type of transducer only has one crystal, if the crystal is damaged, the user will not see an image. In other words, the image, as a whole, is lost. Mechanical transducers have been replaced by more modern transducers in which multiple active elements are arranged in either a straight or a curved line to send out pulses into the body. In these transducers, a defective element will create either a vertical (curvilinear or linear sequential) or horizontal (annular phased-array) band of dropout.

USING A LINEAR ARRAY WITH A DEFECTIVE CRYSTAL

If a sonographer is using a linear sequential (switched)-array transducer and there is a defective PZT crystal, there will be vertical dropout on the screen beneath the active element that has been affected. The image created by a linear sequential probe is rectangular in shape. The pulses sent into the body are fired in groups at different times, but at various locations along the transducer's footprint. These groups of pulses that are transmitted are sent out in a linear fashion and are spaced evenly from each other so that the only part of the image that is affected stems from the scan lines created by the PZT crystal that has been damaged.

ULTRASOUND MACHINE INTEGRITY

Maintaining the integrity of the ultrasound machine ensures that the system is able to deliver dependable diagnostic results. Regular checking enables potential issues to be addressed before there is an impact on imaging and patient care. Verification of ultrasound machine integrity should include the following:

- Check the boot up sequence of the machine. Turn on the machine and observe how the system starts. Ensure that there are no error messages and that the initialization process is smooth.
- Verify that regular calibration is performed for various imaging modes and features. This ensures that the system is always performing up to standards.
- Conduct a thorough assessment of the ultrasound image quality. Evaluate image resolution and overall quality either with a phantom or with other functional testing tools. Document and address any issues as soon as possible.
- Confirm that patient data are stored accurately and are able to be retrieved when necessary. This includes checking that the system is also backing up all relevant data.

ULTRASOUND MACHINE PERFORMANCE MEASUREMENTS

Evaluating ultrasound performance is vital for maintaining the diagnostic accuracy and quality of ultrasound imaging. Assessing parameters such as the dead zone for near-imaging quality, or optimizing the focal zone for image clarity at varying depths contributes to precise diagnoses and optimal patient care. Continuous QA and the use of phantom devices can ensure that the ultrasound system is performing at the highest standard.

DEAD ZONE

The area closest to the transducer is known as the **dead zone**. It involves the region from the transducer to the shallowest point where accurate images appear. Images displayed in this dead zone are typically inaccurate and are therefore unreliable. Shallower dead zones are associated with higher frequency transducers, while deeper dead zones are seen in transducers with a lower frequency. Sonographers should pay special attention to the dead zone because it is possible to misinterpret structures that are near the transducer. If the dead zone is of a significant depth, this can indicate that the backing material has detached, a crystal has cracked, or a long pulse duration. The dead zone can be evaluated with a phantom by assessing the shallowest series of pins.

Focal Zone

The region where ultrasound energy is concentrated is known as the **focal zone**. The ultrasound beam focuses its sound beam in this area and therefore produces the sharpest and clearest images here. Sonographers are able to adjust the focal zone to optimize images at specific depths. A well-optimized focal zone is necessary for ensuring that structures at varying depths can be imaged with precision and detail, aiding in diagnostic accuracy. Phantoms containing targets at different depths can be used to evaluate the focal zone.

Range Accuracy

The ability of an ultrasound system to accurately determine the depth/distance to structures is known as **range accuracy,** or vertical depth calibration. Range accuracy is important because anatomical structures in ultrasound images need to have correct positioning. This contributes to the precision of the ultrasound images produced, ensuring that sonographers can accurately decipher the depth and location of structures on the ultrasound image. In a tissue-mimicking phantom, precision can be evaluated by measuring the distance between two reflected distances and then comparing to the actual known distance.

Axial and Lateral Resolution

A system's ability to distinguish between structures that are closely spaced along the direction of the ultrasound beam is known as **axial resolution**. High axial resolution is paramount for visualizing structures that are close in distance and parallel to the beam. Sonographers should regularly assess axial resolution performance. Phantoms containing targets within close distances on the axial dimension can be used to measure the axial resolution.

Lateral resolution refers to the ability of an ultrasound system to distinguish between structures that are closely spaced together perpendicular to the ultrasound beam. To accurately image structures that are adjacent, high lateral resolution is necessary and should be regularly evaluated. Similar to the axial resolution, phantoms containing targets within close lateral distances can be used to measure the lateral resolution.

Quality Assurance

QUALITY ASSURANCE PROGRAM

Ultrasound labs must have a quality assurance (QA) program. This is necessary to decrease the number of times that a patient must return for additional studies, minimize exams that are not of superior diagnostic quality, and ensure that the ultrasound machine is performing optimally.

This documentation must be available in case of lawsuits to prove that the images and measurement tools are satisfactory. A QA program consists of preventive maintenance by a reputable engineer who can make repairs when necessary. QA must be performed routinely and after an upgrade on a machine. The sonographer plays an important role in making sure that proper QA exams are completed and that a preventive maintenance program is in place.

KEY QUALITY ASSURANCE RESPONSIBILITIES

Incorporating QA checks as a routine operation and keeping comprehensive documentation of each step will result in the optimal quality and reliability of diagnostic ultrasound imaging. The following are specific responsibilities that are commonly included as part of a QA program:

- **Daily checks**—Implementing a daily routine is necessary. Before any patient interaction, a QA check should be performed. This includes ensuring equipment functionality, assessing transducer integrity, and verifying calibration.
- **Image uniformity**—Regularly assess image uniformity and ensure consistency with brightness and resolution across the entire scanning field. Any inconsistencies should be documented and promptly addressed to ensure the quality of diagnostic imaging.
- **Transducer checks**—Routine inspections should be performed for any signs of wear and tear on crystal arrays, cables, and connectors.
- **Doppler performance**—It is imperative to conduct regular checks of Doppler performance, ensuring proper blood flow visualization and velocity measurements. Having consistent Doppler readings ensures optimal performance and diagnostic quality.
- **Recordkeeping**—Not only is it important to perform QA checks, but also to develop a comprehensive recordkeeping system. This serves as a historical record of each QA check, as well as the date, time, and important observations. Documentation of QA checks should also align with industry- and facility-specific guidelines, ensuring compliance and commitment to upholding professional standards.

TESTING WITH TISSUE-MIMICKING PHANTOMS

DOPPLER FLOW PHANTOM

Quality assurance (QA) should play a crucial role in every ultrasound department to help verify that every system offers patients the best image quality possible.

Ultrasound Doppler flow phantoms can assess all Doppler methods, which include color, continuous-wave Doppler, pulsed-wave Doppler, and power Doppler imaging. These devices are used to mimic the cardiovascular system while pumping a substance that is similar to blood. They can represent blood traveling through a vessel with continuous- or pulsed-wave properties and known velocities. Along with the velocities measured, the sensitivities can also be tracked. These systems are used not only for QA purposes, but also for teaching the flow patterns associated with various blood vessels. For example, nonpulsatile or pulsatile flow patterns can be demonstrated as part of a skills lab for new sonographers and physicians.

SLICE THICKNESS PHANTOM

The elevational resolution is best determined with a slice thickness phantom. Slice thickness phantoms contain structures that are similar to soft tissue found in the human body. Elevational resolution pertains to the actual slice thickness of the ultrasound beam. In order to define small cystic components within certain depths of the phantom, the slice thickness must be very thin. When the cystic elements are not discerned at specific depths, it means that there is a wider slice thickness of the ultrasound beam. This occurs when the slice thickness is wider than the cyst; therefore, the return signal includes echoes of the soft tissue on either side of the structure being imaged at the same depth. Thicker slices tend to degrade the image detail or resolution. When this takes place, fluid-filled components may not be visualized at all or may look as if they are filled in.

TISSUE-MIMICKING PHANTOM

Tissue-equivalent phantoms were developed to mimic the properties of soft tissue found in human patients. The speed of ultrasound is only affected by the medium it is passing through. It is important to note that tissue-equivalent phantoms are constructed to exhibit a speed-of-sound, echogenicity, and scattering environment that is similar to soft tissue. A sonographer is not able to adjust the speed of the ultrasound waves. Ultrasound travels at different speeds through various tissue types. Sound travels at an average speed of 1,540 m/s in soft tissue. This can also be expressed as 1.54 km/s or 1.54 mm/μs. Ultrasound travels slowest in gases, quicker in liquids, and fastest in solids. A tissue-equivalent phantom is used to calibrate ultrasound systems because the embedded material has known acoustic properties. These phantoms contain objects that represent solid and cystic masses and materials that demonstrate various reflective properties. Grayscale can be evaluated with this phantom along with multifocus transducers. Phantoms can include small structures that are very similar to cysts and solid masses.

STATISTICAL PARAMETERS

Statistical parameter concepts are paramount in diagnostic testing and evaluation. These include sensitivity, specificity, accuracy, positive predictive value, and negative predictive value.

Sensitivity measures the ability of a diagnostic test to **detect disease** or abnormalities. It is also referred to as the **true positive rate** or **recall**. An ultrasound test that is highly sensitive has the ability to accurately identify cases that are truly positive, ensuring that potential issues are not overlooked during diagnostic imaging.

Specificity measures the ability of a diagnostic test to correctly identify individuals who do not have a particular disease. An ultrasound test that is highly specific has the ability to ensure that normal structures are **not mistakenly identified as a disease**. This means that there are very few false positives, reducing the likelihood for patients to undergo unnecessary testing or treatments.

Accuracy refers to **the overall correctness** of a diagnostic test. It considers both **true positives** and **true negatives.** Ultrasound accuracy is crucial for providing complete and reliable diagnostic information.

Positive predictive value measures the probability that individuals with positive test results **actually have the condition**. It is important in assessing whether detected abnormalities during an ultrasound study are clinically significant.

Negative predictive value measures the probability that individuals with negative test results **truly do not have the condition**. It is relevant in ultrasound to assess whether a normal finding is truly indicative of the absence of disease.

ARDMS Practice Test

Want to take this practice test in an online interactive format? Check out the online resources page, which includes interactive practice questions and much more:
mometrix.com/resources719/ardmssonoprin

1. Sonographers should be aware of work-related musculoskeletal disorders. Best practice while scanning is to avoid abducting the arm more than how many degrees?

    a. 50
    b. 90
    c. 30
    d. 40

2. Which action demonstrates best practice during ultrasound exams regarding the ALARA principle?

    a. The exposure time should be extended during the exam.
    b. Use the lowest possible output power that provides a diagnostic image.
    c. Use the lowest possible gain.
    d. Ensure that the time gain compensation (TGC) is within acceptable limits.

3. Which type of cavitation is the MOST concerning cause of bioeffects?

    a. Transient
    b. Absorption
    c. Stable
    d. Thermal

4. Assuming an unfocused ultrasound beam, the American Institute of Ultrasound in Medicine's "Statement on Mammalian Biological Effects of Ultrasound In Vivo" has confirmed that no bioeffects have been noted when the spatial pulse temporal average (SPTA) intensity is less than which value?

    a. 1 mW/cm^2
    b. 100 W/cm^2
    c. 1 W/cm^2
    d. 100 mW/cm^2

5. A sonographer notices that the mechanical index (MI) is too high during an ultrasound. What would be the MOST appropriate modification that the sonographer can make?
   a. Decrease receiver gain.
   b. Increase period.
   c. Decrease the output power.
   d. Decrease the frequency of the transducer.

6. Select the technique that will generate the LEAST amount of exposure to the patient.
   a. Spectral Doppler
   b. Color flow Doppler
   c. Grayscale
   d. M-mode

7. When a vibrating string or fluid pump is used to test system performance, what parameter is being tested?
   a. Dead zone
   b. Doppler velocities
   c. Contrast resolution
   d. Grayscale sensitivity

8. A tissue-equivalent phantom is used to ensure the efficiency of the ultrasound machine. Choose the resolution that is NOT tested with this phantom.
   a. Temporal
   b. Contrast
   c. Axial
   d. Horizontal

9. Which performance check describes the ability of the ultrasound machine to correctly visualize signals that are weaker than others?
   a. Accuracy
   b. Specificity
   c. Reliability
   d. Sensitivity

10. What is the name of the recent technological advancement that is used on tissues such as the liver, breast, prostate, and thyroid to assess the stiffness of tissue or to better assess lesions?
    a. Contrast-enhanced ultrasound
    b. Fusion imaging
    c. Elastography
    d. Harmonics

11. Which choice is NOT a true statement regarding this filling defect within the gallbladder?

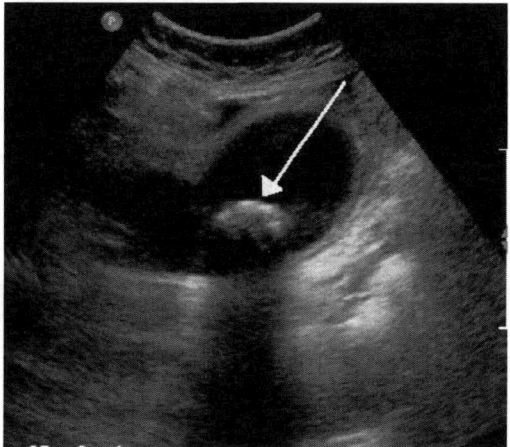

   a. The filling defect displays a significant amount of attenuation.
   b. It has created an enhancement artifact.
   c. It has created a shadowing artifact.
   d. Regions deeper than the filling defect are obscured.

12. Which type of artifact appears echogenic and stems from gas bubbles as they vibrate due to the interaction with the ultrasound beam?
   a. Ring-down artifact
   b. Edge shadow
   c. Crosstalk
   d. Slice thickness

13. What is the fundamental reason that the power and intensity of the ultrasound beam diminish as it travels through tissue?
   a. Absorption
   b. Cavitation
   c. Obstruction
   d. Acoustic impedance

14. Select the modification that the sonographer can make to decrease the amount of attenuation as the ultrasound beam travels through tissues.
   a. Increase the imaging depth.
   b. Increase the frequency of the transducer.
   c. Decrease the output power.
   d. Decrease the frequency of the transducer.

15. Choose the ultrasound system function that enables the sonographer to adapt to the amount of attenuation that occurs with increasing depth.
   a. Focusing
   b. Receiver gain
   c. TGC
   d. Output power

16. Assume that a sound beam is traveling in soft tissue. Calculate the attenuation coefficient if the frequency is 12 MHz.
   a. 12 dB/cm
   b. 6 dB/cm
   c. 8 dB/cm
   d. 10 dB/cm

17. What is NOT a component of attenuation?
   a. Reflection
   b. Scattering
   c. Resolution
   d. Absorption

18. Impedance is NOT influenced by which component?
   a. The frequency of the transducer
   b. Density
   c. Propagation speed
   d. Stiffness

19. For reflection to take place, which situation must exist?
   a. The border of two different tissues must have different impedances.
   b. There must be little difference of the impedances at soft-tissue boundaries.
   c. Normal incidence and identical impedances must be present.
   d. Oblique incidence must occur.

20. While assuming continuous wave (CW) ultrasound, what is the duty factor (DF)?
   a. 0.2%
   b. 1%
   c. 0%
   d. 100%

21. What will happen to the duty factor (DF) if the system increases the pulse repetition frequency (PRF)?
   a. DF remains the same.
   b. DF increases.
   c. DF is not related to PRF.
   d. DF decreases.

22. The best axial resolution will be apparent if the sonographer performs an exam with a transducer that has which characteristic?
   a. Longer pulse length
   b. Longer wavelength
   c. Shorter pulse length
   d. More ringing in the pulse

23. Lateral resolution will be improved if the sonographer performs which operation?
   a. Decreases the scanning depth
   b. Increases the number of focal zones
   c. Maximizes the output power
   d. Uses a lower frequency

24. Which action will NOT increase (or improve) temporal resolution?
   a. Increase the imaging depth.
   b. Decrease the number of focal zones.
   c. Use a sector size that is narrow.
   d. Use a low line density.

25. Which name describes how the angles of the incident and transmission beams are related to the speed of the two media?
   a. Bernoulli's principle
   b. Curie point
   c. Huygens' principle
   d. Snell's law

26. What can be done when investigating a possible kidney stone to better demonstrate shadowing from the stone when using a 3 MHz probe?
   a. Position the focal point deeper than the stone.
   b. Increase the amount of gain.
   c. Increase the frequency to 5 MHz.
   d. Decrease the output power of the system.

27. If the frequency is doubled, what effect will this have on the wavelength?
   a. It will remain the same.
   b. It doubles.
   c. It increases by a factor of 1.54.
   d. It is halved.

28. Which part of the transducer is necessary to reduce the amount of ringing of the piezoelectric (PZT) crystal?
   a. Matching layer
   b. Backing material
   c. Transducer housing
   d. Wire

29. A given frequency of sound is 4.5 MHz, and it has a wavelength of 0.8 mm. How thick should a manufacturer design the matching layer of a transducer in this scenario?
   a. 0.4 mm
   b. 0.16 mm
   c. 0.2 mm
   d. 0.6 mm

30. A sonographer is performing a renal ultrasound. Which transducer frequency will generate the slowest speed of sound?
   a. All frequencies will travel at the same speed in the same tissue.
   b. 2 MHz
   c. 4.5 MHz
   d. 7 MHz

31. Transducers used in image production will have which characteristics?
   a. High Q-factor, wide bandwidth
   b. Low Q-factor, wide bandwidth
   c. Low Q-factor, narrow bandwidth
   d. High Q-factor, narrow bandwidth

32. Which transducer produced the shape of this image?

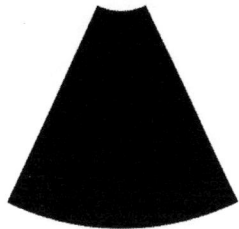

   a. Linear sequential array
   b. Vector array
   c. Annular phased array
   d. Convex array

33. This malfunction takes place in which kind of transducer?

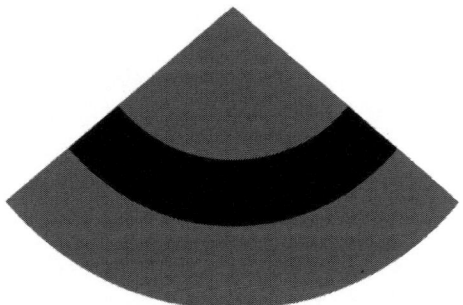

a. Linear sequential array
b. Annular phased array
c. Convex sequential array
d. Mechanical

34. Which statement is NOT true of a linear phased array transducer?

a. The footprint tends to be small.
b. It can alter the number of focal zones and the depth.
c. The image is a rectangle.
d. It uses electronic steering.

35. Select the type of transducer that enables multi-focusing while being steered mechanically.

a. Annular phased array
b. Mechanical
c. Linear sequential array
d. Convex sequential array

36. If the diameter of the PZT crystal is 13 mm, which sentence describes the sound wave's diameter in the Fresnel zone?

a. The sound beam will be half of the diameter of the crystal in the Fresnel zone.
b. 13 mm
c. 26 mm
d. The sound wave narrows as it leaves the transducer.

37. The amount of divergence that occurs in the far field is determined by the sound wave's frequency and which component?

a. Line density
b. Focal zone depth
c. Diameter of the crystal
d. Speed

38. Select the type of transducer that produces an image that takes on the shape of a parallelogram when it is electronically steered.
   a. Linear phased array
   b. Linear sequential array
   c. Annular phased array
   d. Convex array

39. Choose the type of transducer that lacks range resolution.
   a. Phased array
   b. Annular array
   c. Continuous wave (CW)
   d. Linear sequential array

40. In this phased array transducer, what direction will the beam be steered?

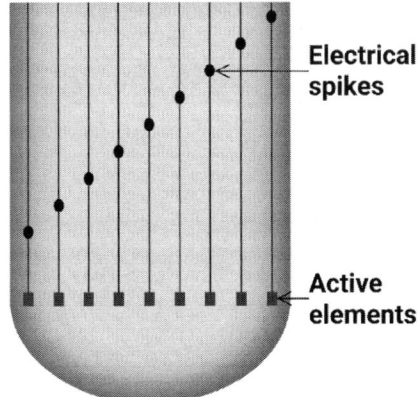

   a. 45 degrees to the right
   b. Slightly to the left
   c. Slightly to the right
   d. 45 degrees to the left

41. What configuration is necessary to focus the ultrasound wave in a linear phased array transducer?
   a. Electronic slope
   b. Dynamic aperture
   c. PZT crystals
   d. Electronic curve

42. Which parameter is decreased by the ultrasound machine to evade the possibility of range ambiguity when the imaging depth is increased?
   a. Number of scan lines
   b. Pulse repetition frequency (PRF)
   c. Pulse repetition period (PRP)
   d. Persistence

43. Which phrase does NOT describe an effect that focusing has on the ultrasound beam?
   a. A bigger focal zone
   b. Enhanced near zone resolution
   c. Diminished lateral resolution of the far zone
   d. Results in a shorter near zone

44. Select the answer that best describes how B-mode will typically display blood vessels?
   a. Hyperechoic
   b. Isogenic
   c. Anechoic
   d. Heterogeneous

45. How deep is a reflector if the go-return time of a sound wave is 39 μs?
   a. 2 cm
   b. 3 cm
   c. 5 cm
   d. 6 cm

46. Why does grayscale imaging require the use of pulsed wave ultrasound?
   a. To optimize penetration
   b. To optimize temporal resolution
   c. To determine the bandwidth
   d. To determine the depth of the reflector

47. Which system function is modified if the ultrasound user adjusts the receiver gain?
   a. Demodulation
   b. Reject
   c. Amplification
   d. Compression

48. When M-mode is employed during an echocardiogram, what information is depicted on the display?
   a. Depth and amplitude
   b. Time and frequency
   c. Amplitude, motion, and time
   d. Depth, time, and frequency

49. If an ultrasound image displays high contrast, what correlates with the dynamic range?
   a. Wide dynamic range
   b. Narrow dynamic range
   c. No effect on the range
   d. A display of many shades of gray

50. Which component of the ultrasound wave increases if the sonographer increases the output gain?

   a. Pulse duration
   b. Frequency
   c. Noise
   d. Intensity

51. What is the name of the frequency used in tissue harmonics that is responsible for image production?

   a. Fundamental frequency
   b. Spatial compounding
   c. Overall gain
   d. Harmonic frequency

52. Which one of the following applies when using tissue harmonics to image the gallbladder?

   a. Use of lower frequencies
   b. Use of higher frequencies
   c. Decreased lateral resolution
   d. Increased reverberation artifacts

53. Which type of zoom is a preprocessing function that provides more pixels in the region of interest, resulting in superior spatial resolution?

   a. Temporal resolution
   b. Read zoom
   c. Write zoom
   d. Read magnification

54. Which control on the ultrasound system should be adjusted if it is necessary to reduce the amount of noise in the image?

   a. Reject
   b. Amplification
   c. Compression
   d. Demodulation

55. During a renal ultrasound, the sonographer finds it necessary to adjust controls on the ultrasound system to improve the image. What CANNOT be adjusted by the operator?

   a. Output power
   b. Amplitude
   c. Frequency
   d. Speed

56. What control offers better visualization of fibroids by increasing far field penetration and resolution?
    a. Persistence
    b. Spatial compounding
    c. Coded excitation
    d. Elastography

57. Which control can a sonographer apply to help delineate a subtle liver mass?
    a. Zoom
    b. Edge enhancement
    c. Fill-in interpolation
    d. Increase the receiver gain

58. Which phrase correctly describes the following ultrasound beam?

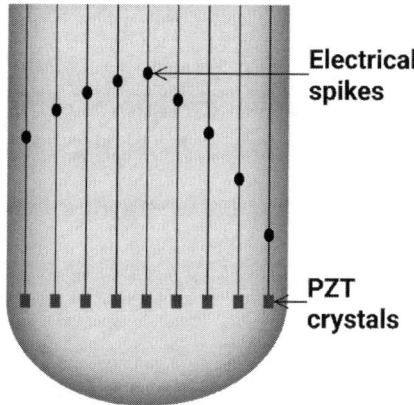

    a. Unfocused, no steering
    b. Focused, steered to the right
    c. Unfocused, steered to the left
    d. Focused, steered to the left

59. What is the name of the approach to image production in which the reflected ultrasound beam is averaged among multiple frequencies to lessen the effects of noise and speckle in the image?
    a. Spatial compounding
    b. Tissue harmonics
    c. Frequency compounding
    d. Temporal compounding

60. What is a function of the receiver?
    a. It shapes the ultrasound beam.
    b. It controls the collaboration of the synergy of the ultrasound components.
    c. It stores images and video clips.
    d. It changes and displays the signal sent from the transducer to the monitor.

61. What is the correct order in which the receiver functions during image production?
   a. Amplification, compensation, compression, demodulation, reject
   b. Amplification, reject, demodulation, compensation, compression
   c. Amplification, demodulation, compression, reject, compensation
   d. Amplification, compression, demodulation, reject, compensation

62. Preprocessing functions occur before the data reaches which component of the ultrasound system?
   a. Pulser
   b. Scan converter
   c. Receiver
   d. Beam former

63. Which phrase describes the scenario in which persistence will be best used?
   a. When persistence cannot be adjusted by the user
   b. During the interrogation of rapid blood flow
   c. During the interrogation of slow blood flow
   d. When more noise is desired during image production

64. When using 3D ultrasound, what is the name of the smallest element of the picture that is generated?
   a. Pixel
   b. Voxel
   c. Byte
   d. Bit

65. Digital imaging systems require which component to link the ultrasound system and the archiving network?
   a. BIT
   b. RIS
   c. PACS
   d. DICOM

66. Which component enables facilities that use digital imaging to archive and share the images of exams performed in the department?
   a. RIS
   b. PACS
   c. BIT
   d. DICOM

67. Which list describes the progression in which a signal moves through an ultrasound machine?
   a. Scan converter, transducer, display, receiver
   b. Transducer, scan converter, display, receiver
   c. Scan converter, receiver, display, transducer
   d. Transducer, receiver, scan converter, display

68. Which choice will optimize the spatial resolution?
   a. 1,500 × 1,500 analog
   b. 200 × 200 pixels
   c. 800 × 800 pixels
   d. 300 × 300 digital

69. Which system control was used to create the following image?

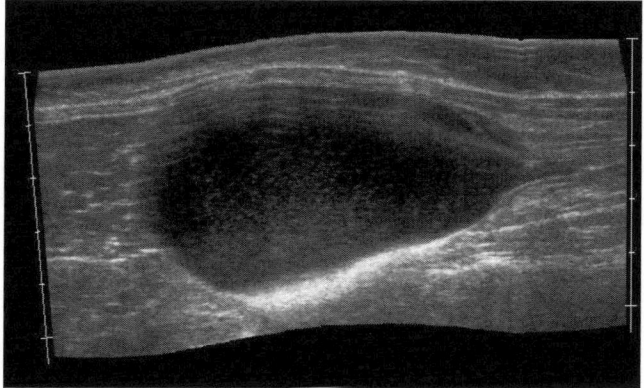

   a. Elastography
   b. Color Doppler
   c. Extended field of view (EFOV)
   d. B-mode

70. Which region is NOT a component of a TGC curve?
   a. Phase quadrature
   b. Knee
   c. Near gain
   d. Slope

71. If 3 bits of memory are available, what is the greatest number of shades of gray that are present in the scan converter?
   a. 4
   b. 8
   c. 16
   d. 32

72. The best contrast resolution will be available with which digital scan converter?

   a. 4 bits
   b. 256 shades of gray
   c. 32 shades of gray
   d. 16 bits

73. Which scanning angles will provide the most significant amount of Doppler shift to measure the peak velocity during a carotid duplex ultrasound?

   a. 0 or 90 degrees
   b. 90 or 180 degrees
   c. 115 or 180 degrees
   d. 0 or 180 degrees

74. Which image demonstrates the correct placement of the gate to obtain the most accurate blood flow velocity measurement?

a.
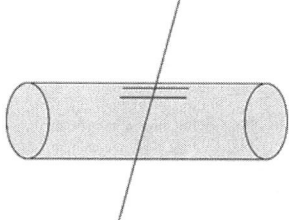

b.
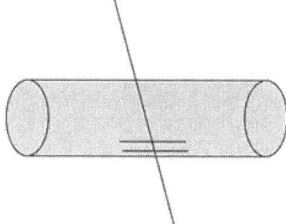

c.
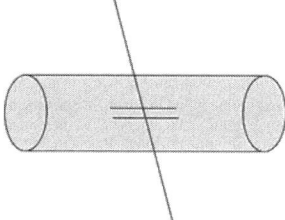

d.
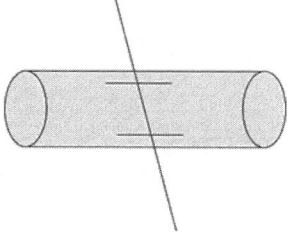

75. Which of the following represents the approximate diameter reduction of the internal carotid artery (ICA) when evaluating the spectral waveform and peak systolic velocity (PSV) and end-diastolic velocity (EDV) information?

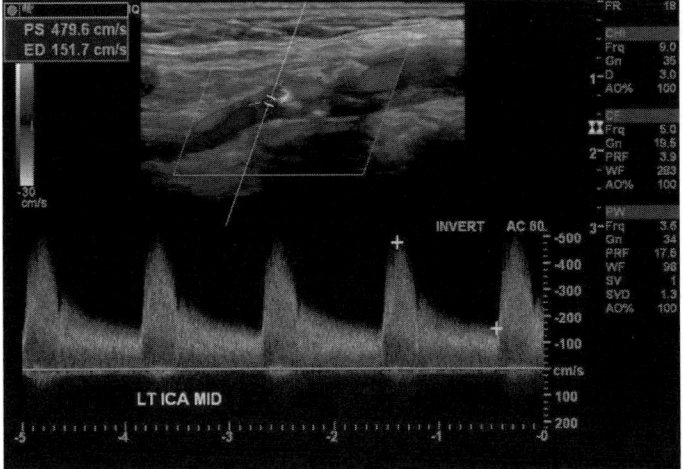

   a. 25–49%
   b. 50–79%
   c. 80–99%
   d. 100%

76. If a sonographer asks a patient to take in a deep breath and hold it, what is the result of venous blood flow in the legs?
   a. The flow becomes turbulent.
   b. The flow rate decreases.
   c. The flow rate increases.
   d. The flow becomes pulsatile.

77. Which statement is true regarding these images?

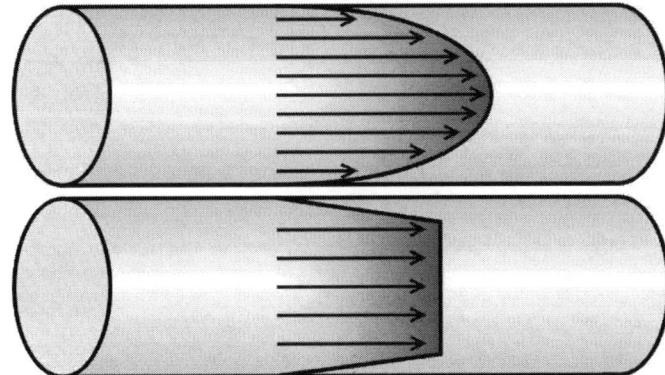

   a. The blood flow represented in these vessels is considered to be laminar flow.
   b. The Reynolds number in these vessels is likely more than 2,000.
   c. The blood flow represented in these vessels will be chaotic.
   d. Eddy currents will likely be present within these blood vessels.

78. If a carotid duplex exam is performed on a patient with a 7 MHz and a 14 MHz transducer, which transducer will display a Doppler shift that is greater?
   a. The 14 MHz transducer
   b. The Doppler shift is the same with both transducers.
   c. The 7 MHz transducer
   d. The Doppler shift cannot be identified with this information.

79. Which step CANNOT be used to correct the imaging error seen in the following tracing of the external carotid artery (ECA)?

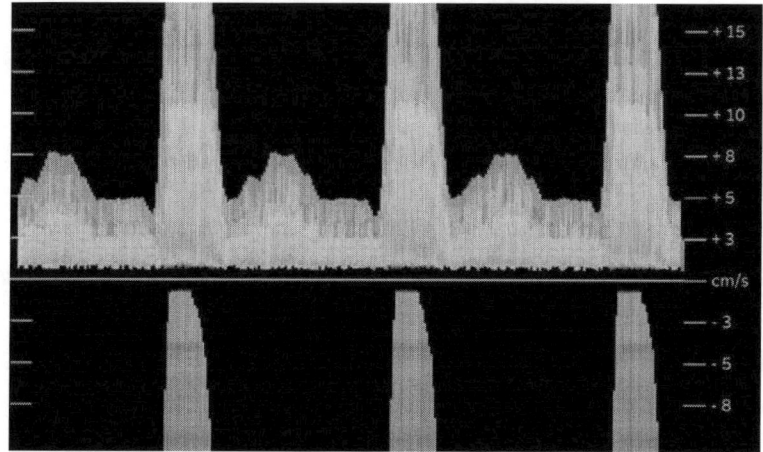

   a. Switch to a lower frequency transducer.
   b. Move the baseline down.
   c. Reposition the gate to a location that is deeper.
   d. Increase the pulse repetition frequency (PRF) to its maximum value.

80. While using pulsed wave Doppler, the sonographer believes that the measurements are not accurate. After switching to a 4.5 MHz continuous wave (CW) Doppler at a depth of 5 cm, what will the maximum velocity cap be?
   a. There will not be a maximum velocity cap with CW Doppler.
   b. 45 cm/s
   c. 150 cm/s
   d. This cannot be determined with the given information.

81. What will the aliasing frequency be if a renal artery duplex exam is performed at a depth of 6 cm, the length of the sample volume is 0.50 mm, and the pulse repetition frequency (PRF) is 8 kHz with the Doppler frequency at 3.5 MHz?
   a. 3.5 MHz
   b. 8 kHz
   c. 7 MHz
   d. 4 kHz

82. Which statement is NOT true concerning color Doppler?
   a. Doppler frequency shift is reached with the use of the autocorrelation method.
   b. Aliasing may occur when using color Doppler.
   c. Color Doppler is a reliable method to measure the peak systolic and end-diastolic velocities.
   d. Range resolution exists with color Doppler.

83. If a sonographer must interrogate a blood vessel that displays slow flow once color Doppler is applied, what should be done to the pulse repetition frequency (PRF) to improve the visualization of flow?
   a. Adjusting the PRF has no effect.
   b. Decrease the PRF.
   c. Increase the PRF.
   d. Adjusting the PRF will create aliasing.

84. If the red blood cells are traveling away from the transducer, what type of Doppler shift is present?
   a. Negative
   b. Unequivocal
   c. None
   d. Positive

85. A sonographer has access to 10 MHz linear sequential, 7 MHz linear sequential, and 4.5 MHz curved array transducers. If the 10 MHz transducer produces aliasing during a carotid duplex study, what can be done to alleviate this issue if a shallower window did NOT correct the problem?
   a. Switch to the 4.5 MHz curved array transducer.
   b. Neither of the two remaining transducers will resolve this issue.
   c. Switch to the 7 MHz linear sequential transducer.
   d. None of these transducers should be used for carotid duplex exams.

86. If the sonographer does not see any color flow when applied but could see movement of blood cells within the vessel on grayscale imaging, what should the operator assume?
   a. Power Doppler must be used instead.
   b. The angle of incidence is 90 degrees and needs to be changed.
   c. The blood vessel is obstructed.
   d. Maintenance must be called as the color Doppler is not sensitive enough.

87. When using spectral Doppler, the sonographer notices information that correlates with lower velocities missing from the waveform. What control can be modified to demonstrate these velocities?
   a. Wall filter
   b. Scale
   c. Depth
   d. Gain

88. If the Reynolds number is 2,078, what does this suggest?
   a. Plug flow
   b. Laminar flow
   c. Disturbed flow
   d. Turbulent flow

89. The carotid artery is being examined with color Doppler. Which artifact is present if the color appears to be bleeding outside of the vessel when color Doppler is applied?
   a. Clutter
   b. Crosstalk
   c. Ghosting
   d. Aliasing

90. If a sonographer measures the peak systolic velocity (PSV) from the ICA and the spectral window appears filled in with blood moving in various directions, what does this indicate?
   a. Spectral broadening
   b. Patent ICA
   c. The gain is set too high.
   d. Laminar flow

91. The ultrasound operator is attempting to measure the velocity of flow within the femoral artery but is incidentally picking up signals within the femoral vein. Which control on the ultrasound system will enable the sonographer to adjust the position of the gate?
   a. Angle correction
   b. Triplex
   c. Sweep speed
   d. Pulse repetition frequency (PRF)

92. If it is necessary to improve the frame rate during a color Doppler exam, which step is the best action to accomplish this?
   a. Angle the color box.
   b. Decrease the gain.
   c. Increase the depth in which the color box is located.
   d. Decrease the width of the color box.

93. Which operator setting will increase the patient's exposure during a carotid duplex exam?
   a. Increasing the Doppler angle
   b. Increasing the pulse repetition frequency (PRF)
   c. A higher baseline location
   d. Increasing the Doppler gain

94. Which operation will improve the frame rate when using color Doppler to interrogate the ovaries?
   a. Change the color map.
   b. Increase the packet size.
   c. Decrease the packet size.
   d. Adjust the color Doppler gain.

95. Which is NOT a reason a sonographer would choose to use power Doppler during a renal duplex exam?
   a. The velocity of the blood is accurately measured with power Doppler.
   b. Aliasing will not occur with power Doppler.
   c. The sensitivity of power Doppler is greater than that of color Doppler.
   d. The amplitude of the signal is displayed with power Doppler.

96. Aliasing is seen while scanning the femoral artery at a 30-degree angle. Which step will correct this artifact?
   a. Reduce the angle of incidence.
   b. Increase the frequency of the transducer.
   c. Find a window that is deeper.
   d. Increase the pulse repetition frequency (PRF).

97. A sonographer uses the color map during a color Doppler exam of the carotid artery and notices that the colors in the middle of the map appear to be communicating with each other. Which choice best describes this scenario?
   a. Aliasing is present.
   b. The flow in the carotid artery is bidirectional.
   c. The flow in the carotid artery is unidirectional.
   d. The wall filter is set too high.

98. When the screen is sector shaped, what can be modified when color Doppler is used?
   a. Steering of the color box
   b. Size and location of the color box
   c. Shape of the color box
   d. Velocity of the moving red blood cells

99. Which choice will improve the color fill of this blood vessel?

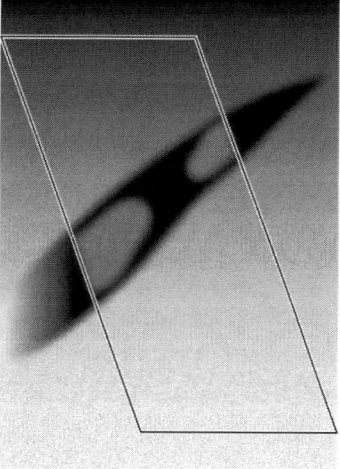

a. Change the steering of the color box.
b. Increase the output power.
c. Change the window so the vessel is shallower.
d. Decrease the color gain.

100. Which choice is NOT an instance of when a sonographer would expect to see spectral broadening?

a. When sampling the velocity within a tight stenosis of the internal carotid artery
b. When sampling the velocity distal to a tight stenosis of the external carotid artery
c. When measuring the velocity within a patent internal carotid artery
d. When sampling the velocity at the bifurcation of the carotid artery

Answer Key and Explanations

1. C: Sonographers should use correct ergonomics to care for their own bodies to prevent work-related musculoskeletal disorders. Roughly 80% of sonographers report having some sort of work injury. Ergonomics is a combination of setting up the room appropriately so the patient and machine can be reached easily. Properly using equipment that reinforces the desired body mechanics to prevent any injuries is also key. This may be something as simple as adjusting the keyboard or monitor to the correct height. One of the most common complaints that a sonographer makes is pain in the shoulder while scanning. It is imperative that the patient is close enough so that the sonographer's arm does not have to be abducted more than 30 degrees. The other choices would not protect the sonographer because they are all angles that are more than 30 degrees.

2. B: Sonographers should always consider ways to practice the ALARA principle. ALARA stands for as low as reasonably achievable, and sonographers can achieve this by using the lowest possible output power that enables a diagnostic image. Keeping the exposure time to a minimum is another effective way of practicing ALARA. The gain can change the brightness (or darkness) of the image, but it has no effect on patient exposure, so the power should always be reduced, if possible, before the gain to reduce exposure to the patient. On the other hand, if an image is too dark, it is best to increase the gain because it will not affect exposure to the patient. Time gain compensation (TGC) enables the sonographer to adjust the amplification of reflections that are located at a greater depth in the body, but it has no effect on the exposure.

3. A: Cavitation is discussed when bioeffects are considered with the interaction of the ultrasound beam and gas bubbles in the human body. Higher temperatures and pressures may cause the gas bubbles within the body to burst; this is known as transient cavitation, which is extremely concerning for harmful bioeffects. When these gas bubbles expand and contract with fluctuations in pressure without rupturing, it is referred to as stable cavitation. There are only two types of cavitation, so absorption and thermal are not viable answers to this question.

4. D: The spatial pulse temporal average (SPTA) is linked with the greatest amount of temperature elevation within tissues. Bioeffects have not been noted when the SPTA intensity was less than 100 mW/cm^2, when the ultrasound beam was unfocused. If the ultrasound beam is focused, then the same principle applies if the intensity is less than 1 W/cm^2. If there is an inquiry regarding the smallest intensity, the answer would be the spatial average temporal average.

5. C: The mechanical index (MI) is a parameter that the user should monitor to help determine if cavitation is expected. If a sonographer notices that the MI is too high during an ultrasound, it is important to decrease the acoustic power of the machine. Another step the sonographer can do to keep the MI lower is to *increase* the frequency of the transducer. The receiver gain has no effect on patient exposure.

The ultrasound operator is not able to adjust the period unless a different transducer is chosen.

6. C: The lowest level of tissue heating occurs when the output intensity of the equipment being used is at its lowest numerical value. Generally, grayscale imaging is the method in which tissue heating will be the lowest. It is typically the highest when pulsed Doppler is being used. M-mode and color flow Doppler tend to fall in the middle of these intensities.

Ultrasound should be used only for clinical exams in which the benefits outweigh the risks. One risk during an exam is an elevation of temperature in tissues exposed to the ultrasound beam. The thermal index (TI) will be highest during an exam with a high-frequency, high-intensity beam. This heating depends on the exposure time and the temperature. Typically, the greatest increase in temperature is witnessed with spectral Doppler exams.

7. B: A vibrating string or fluid pump is used to test Doppler velocities of an ultrasound system. These Doppler phantoms enable the evaluation of particles in motion that mimic blood flowing through blood vessels to determine the accuracy of velocities as well as the resolution at various depths. The dead zone is the region within the first centimeter of the transducer. Contrast resolution and grayscale sensitivity can both be evaluated with a tissue-equivalent phantom.

8. A: A tissue-equivalent phantom (also referred to as a grayscale or tissue-mimicking phantom) is important because it evaluates the sensitivity of the system's grayscale capabilities. This type of phantom can distinguish between shades of gray that are even marginally different, such as in contrast resolution. Axial resolution can also be evaluated with a tissue-equivalent phantom because separate structures that are parallel to the ultrasound wave can be seen individually as one in front of the other. Horizontal resolution is the ability to determine that reflectors are in the proper locations when they are perpendicular and in a horizontal position in relation to the ultrasound beam. Horizontal resolution can also be assessed in a tissue-equivalent phantom. Temporal resolution depends on the frame rate and is not tested with a tissue-equivalent phantom.

9. D: Sensitivity refers to the ability of an ultrasound machine to demonstrate weaker signals. Accuracy is the ability of an exam to diagnose outcomes that are positive and negative. Specificity is when an imaging exam can correctly diagnose results that are normal. Reliability refers to the ability of an exam to produce results that are dependable and consistent.

10. C: Elastography is a recent ultrasound technology that uses sound waves to test the stiffness of tissue or lesions that are being evaluated. Elastography is used most often when evaluating the liver, breast, or prostate or for thyroid disease. Contrast-enhanced ultrasound involves injecting (or giving orally) contrast to help visualize tumors or to evaluate blood vessels. Fusion imaging involves concurrent ultrasound imaging with a previous computed tomography or magnetic resonance imaging scan on a split screen to enhance diagnostic confidence that an area previously mentioned is the same area being evaluated. This can be extremely helpful during ultrasound-guided biopsies. Harmonics are signals that are produced by the patient's body (not the ultrasound system). This technology has been in use for several years.

11. B: In this image, a gallstone (cholelithiasis) is the filling defect that is visualized within the lumen of the gallbladder. Artifacts can offer important information such as shadowing from something that is calcified such as a gallstone, as seen in this instance, or even a kidney stone. This filling defect attenuates a great deal and has created a shadowing artifact, which is the hypoechoic area that is seen underneath the gallstone. The regions deep to the filling defect are obscured due to the shadowing. The opposite of a shadowing artifact is one that is known as an enhancement artifact. This type of artifact can also be advantageous for sonographers and interpreting physicians because it appears as a hyperechoic region underneath a structure that demonstrates a lower attenuation rate such as a cyst or the gallbladder.

12. A: A ring-down artifact (also known as a comet-tail artifact) occurs when the reflectors are parallel to the ultrasound beam; it looks like an echogenic line. An edge shadow is due to the refraction of the sound beam; it appears like a dark shadow that extends deep to a curved structure. Crosstalk occurs only with spectral Doppler as a mirror image artifact in which blood flow looks as if it is moving in two directions. A slice-thickness artifact can degrade image details if the slice thickness of the ultrasound beam is wider than the target. When this takes place, fluid-filled components may not be visualized at all or they may look like they are filled in because the return signal is including soft tissue on either side of the cyst at the same depth.

13. A: Attenuation is a term that describes the weakening of the ultrasound beam as it passes through tissues. This weakening applies to the power, amplitude, and intensity of the beam. The fundamental cause of attenuation is absorption because the energy of the beam is changed to heat. Cavitation refers to the possibility of bioeffects occurring during an exam. Obstruction is not a term that is related to attenuation, and acoustic impedance is the hindrance of sound as it passes through a medium, which affects the reflection of a sound wave.

14. D: The amount of attenuation will be decreased if the sonographer decreases the frequency of the transducer. Absorption is one of the main causes of attenuation, and attenuation increases when the sonographer increases the frequency of the transducer, making this choice incorrect. The distance that the sound wave travels has a direct impact on attenuation, so increasing the imaging depth will increase attenuation (not decrease as asked in this instance). Decreasing the output power creates more attenuation because the ultrasound wave is not as strong.

15. C: Time gain compensation (TGC) is a function of the ultrasound system that allows the sonographer to compensate for the weaker signals (attenuation) as the sound waves travel further into the body. This control will allow for uniform brightness when set correctly because the user can adjust at specific depths when necessary. Receiver gain will implement a change to the entire image and not just at certain depths. Focusing will create a beam that is narrower at the focal point, enhancing the resolution at this point. Adjusting the output power will either increase or decrease the energy of the ultrasound beam, creating an entire image that is brighter or darker and affects patient exposure.

16. B: The attenuation coefficient describes how the intensity of the ultrasound beam decreases when considering the distance and frequency of the ultrasound wave. The attenuation coefficient units are decibels per centimeter (dB/cm). Attenuation occurs because of reflection, scattering, and absorption of the sound beam's energy. Frequency is directly related to scattering and absorption, so we can assume that frequency is also directly related to the attenuation coefficient. The equation that can be used to calculate this is as follows:

Attenuation coefficient (dB/cm) $= \frac{\text{frequency (MHz)}}{2} = \frac{12}{2} = 6$ dB/cm.

17. C: Resolution refers to image quality and is not a component of attenuation. Recall that as a sound beam passes through the body, the intensity is diminished (as are the amplitude and power). Three components contribute to the attenuation of a sound beam: reflection, scattering, and absorption. Reflection occurs if a part of the sound beam is sent back toward the transducer. Specular and diffuse are two types of reflections. Specular reflection takes place when there is a smooth boundary such as looking in a mirror. This portion of the beam, however, does not return directly back to the transducer but at an angle. Diffuse reflections take place at a boundary that is not smooth and tends to reflect in various directions known as backscatter. Scattering is the second component of attenuation that occurs when the energy tends to travel in many directions. One cannot predict where scattering will take place, and an ultrasound beam with a higher frequency will demonstrate more scatter. Absorption is the third component of attenuation; it describes when the energy of the ultrasound wave is changed to heat.

18. A: Impedance can be defined as the interference of the transmission of sound as it moves through tissue. Impedance is the product of the medium's density and propagation speed of the medium, so if the density and speed increase, impedance will also increase. Acoustic impedance is a calculation that has an impact on the amount of reflection that occurs. If two tissues have the same impedance, all of the sound will be transmitted. If two tissue types have vastly different impedances, the majority of the sound will be reflected. Stiffness has a direct relationship to speed, therefore also influencing impedance. The frequency of the transducer does not influence the impedance because impedance is related only to the medium.

19. A: Reflection takes places when some of the energy of the sound wave is averted back toward the transducer. Reflection will occur only if the borders of two different tissues have different impedances; otherwise, transmission occurs. Recall that the incident intensity is the intensity of a sound beam as it leaves the transducer prior to coming into contact with tissue. The transmitted intensity is the forward propagation of the intensity of the incident beam after hitting that boundary. Normal incidence is when the incident sound beam comes into contact with the boundary at a 90-degree angle. During diagnostic imaging, there are few differences in the impedance of soft-tissue boundaries; therefore, more than 99% of the incident beam will be transmitted. To summarize, with normal incidence and identical impedances of the media, all of the incident beam's intensity will be transmitted. Keep in mind that the incident and transmitted intensities must always equal 100%. Oblique incidence and reflection (or transmission) are hard to conclude because they tend to be complex.

20. D: Duty factor (DF) is the percentage of time that an ultrasound system is imparting sound waves. For continuous wave (CW) systems, the DF is 100% because a signal is always being sent (but is unable to generate an ultrasound image because images can be created only with pulsed waves). A DF of 0% means that a system is not generating a pulse. Recall that the maximum value for DF of a CW sound beam is 100% and the minimum value is 0%. Pulses are necessary to create images, and the typical DF for imaging is 0.2%, which is for pulsed wave systems.

21. B: The DF is the percentage of time that a transducer is actively transmitting a signal. DF is a calculation that has no units; rather, it will be expressed as a percentage. The ranges of DF for clinical imaging fall into the 0.002–0.005 range or 0.2%–0.5%. These ranges of diagnostic ultrasound indicate that a small percentage of time is spent transmitting a pulse and a large percentage of time is used for listening. The DF is calculated by the following equation:

$$DF = \frac{\text{pulse duration}}{\text{pulse repetition period (PRP)}} \times 100.$$

The pulse repetition frequency (PRF) is defined as the number of pulses sent into the body in one second. DF and PRF are both affected by the imaging depth and will have a direct relationship with each other, which makes incorrect. The PRF is inversely related to the depth of the object being studied, as is the DF. As the depth decreases, the PRF increases because new pulses are constantly being sent because the listening time is shorter. If the depth increases, the PRF decreases (as will the DF) because there is more listening time, so the return time has to be greater. If the PRF increases, DF also increases because the amount of time the system is "on," or transmitting a pulse, increases.

22. C: Axial resolution is enhanced when shorter pulse lengths are being produced. Axial resolution is considered superior to lateral resolution in diagnostic imaging because ultrasound pulses tend to be shorter than the width of the beam. It should be noted that an increase in focusing tends to degrade axial resolution because the result is a longer pulse length. More ringing in the pulse indicates that more cycles are present in the pulse, and, therefore, the axial resolution will not be improved.

23. B: Lateral resolution depends on the width of the ultrasound beam. It will be improved if the sonographer increases the number of focal zones while scanning a patient because this is the narrowest portion of the beam (focus). Lateral resolution is enhanced at the focus. This action will, however, slow down the frame rate. Lateral resolution (also referred to as angular, azimuthal, and transverse) describes the capability of the system to demonstrate separate reflectors when they are perpendicular to the ultrasound beam. If the user decreases the scanning depth, this will improve the lateral resolution only when it is the focal point as well, but unlike axial resolution, the lateral resolution does change with the imaging depth. The output power will not affect the lateral resolution. Switching to a lower frequency will generate a wider beam that degrades the lateral resolution.

24. A: Temporal resolution describes the capability of the ultrasound machine to image in real time and is dependent on the frame rate. The frame rate depends on the imaging depth and how many pulses are in each frame. One of the most common steps performed to increase temporal resolution is to decrease the depth during an ultrasound exam. A structure that is located deeper in the body will require a greater time of flight because the system is transmitting the pulses into the body and then back to the transducer to be processed. This additional time will decrease the frame rate and temporal resolution. If the user needs to increase temporal resolution, the scanning depth should always remain as shallow as possible, so there is less time required to process a signal. If a user increases the imaging depth, temporal resolution decreases (slows down) because it takes more time for the signal to return to the system. In other words, an increase in depth decreases the frame rate. When temporal resolution decreases, the operator will notice a lag in the image.

25. D: Refraction is the bending of a sound beam when it travels from one medium to another. Two conditions must apply for refraction to take place in a clinical setting:

1. There must be an oblique angle of incidence
2. The two media must be traveling at different speeds because refraction cannot take place if the media have identical speeds.

Clinically, an ultrasound beam will bend slightly only at various tissue interfaces. Bone tends to create larger refraction angles because the speed of ultrasound in bone is faster than the speed of sound in soft tissues. Snell's law is used to calculate refraction, and the following equation may be used:

$$\frac{\sin(\text{angle of transmission})}{\sin(\text{angle of incidence})} = \frac{\text{speed in medium 2}}{\text{speed in medium 1}}$$

Bernoulli's principle refers to the correlation between velocity and pressure in a fluid. The Curie point refers to the temperature at which polarization of the active element takes place. Huygens' principle explains the hourglass appearance of an ultrasound beam.

26. C: A sonographer can improve the resolution in what appears to be kidney stones (nephrolithiasis) by two methods. If stones are suspected, but distal acoustic shadowing is not clearly identified with a 3 MHz probe, the sonographer can increase the frequency as high as it will go. Higher frequency transducers will create an ultrasound beam that is narrower. If the ultrasound wave is wider than the stone, the beam picks up signals from either side of the stone, and the shadow may not be visualized as well or at all. In this case, perhaps the operator can bump the frequency all the way up to 5 MHz. Another adjustment that can be performed to create a narrow beam is to place the focal point at the depth of the kidney stones. The gain and output power will not affect visualization of the stones.

27. D: The definition of wavelength is the length of one cycle. Wavelength will be displayed in any unit of distance, and the usual range in diagnostic ultrasound imaging is 0.1–0.8 mm. The medium and the sound source are factors that determine the wavelength. Wavelength is not a control on the ultrasound system that a sonographer can change; rather, wavelength changes when changing transducers that have a different frequency. To calculate the wavelength of a sound beam in soft tissue, the following formula can be used:

$$\text{wavelength in soft tissue} = \frac{1.54}{\text{frequency}}.$$

Using this formula, one can visualize the inverse relationship between the wavelength and the frequency, and if the frequency is doubled, the wavelength will be halved, making the only correct choice.

28. B: The backing material is the component of the transducer that will diminish the time (and length) that the PZT crystal is ringing. This layer is attached to the back of the active element to control any excess vibrations. Longer pulses tend to create images with poor axial resolution. Axial resolution will be improved with a shorter pulse length and duration that the crystal is excited. The backing material is also referred to as the damping element and has an impedance that is similar to PZT while retaining much of the energy of the sound (absorption). The matching layer is situated between the patient and the PZT crystal, and it is there to decrease the impedance at the boundary of the skin and the transducer face. The transducer housing is to protect the patient and the user from electrical shock. The wire couples the PZT crystals and the ultrasound machine.

29. C: The purpose of the matching layer is to enable the ultrasound energy to make a smooth transition from the transducer into the patient's body by curbing the reflections at the skin. Ultrasound gel also helps transmit the sound beam into the body by eliminating the air gap. The thickness of the transducer's matching layer should be one-quarter of the wavelength of the sound beam. In this instance, the length of the wavelength is $0.8(1/4) = 0.2$.

30. A: The frequency of sound will travel at the same speed when traveling through the same medium. The speed of sound does not rely on the transducer frequency, only the medium (which is renal tissue in this example). The speed of sound cannot be changed by the operator, so all three frequencies will travel at the same speed if they are within the same tissue. The speed will change only if they are all located in different types of tissues.

31. B: Ultrasound labs use pulsed wave imaging transducers that contain backing material. Backing material (also referred to as damping material) is used to optimize the axial resolution. This is accomplished by attaching a mix of epoxy resin and tungsten particles to the back of the active element or PZT crystal. Using backing material will decrease the sensitivity of the transducer, create a wide bandwidth (range of operating frequencies), and be referred to as having a low quality (Q) factor. The Q-factor refers to the authenticity of the beam. Non-imaging probes do not contain backing material, which creates a narrow bandwidth. Non-imaging probes, for example, CW Doppler and therapeutic ultrasound transducers, are known as having a high Q-factor, which displays a narrow bandwidth.

32. D: The image shape in this question is referred to as a blunted sector. It resembles the classic sector-shaped image at greater depths, but the difference lies at the top of the image. The indentation is associated with the curvature of the transducer face in convex array probes. A linear sequential array produces an image in the shape of a rectangle. A vector array transducer produces an image that is in the shape of a trapezoid. An annular phased array transducer produces images that are sector shaped with a sharp point at the top.

33. B: This image demonstrates an image in which the midportion is lost due to a horizontal band of dropout, which is demonstrated by the black band. The user will still be able to see the rest of the image that is not within this horizontal band. This malfunction has taken place in one of the rings of an annular phased array transducer. If an element malfunctions in either a linear sequential array or a convex sequential array transducer, the result will be a vertical band of dropout beneath the damaged crystal. Recall that a mechanical transducer only has one active element, so if this crystal is damaged, the sonographer will not see an image at all when attempting to scan.

34. C: There are many advantages of using any transducer with phased array technology. Linear phased array probes have small footprints, enabling easier intercostal scanning. Another advantage is that the sonographer can electronically focus the ultrasound beam at all depths during an exam. Focusing can be optimized regardless of the depth of the anatomical structure being interrogated. Steering is also controlled electronically. With linear phased array transducers, the part that touches the patient is flat, but the beam is sent into the body in a nonlinear fashion, creating an image that is sector shaped. In other words, the pulses can also reach structures in the body that are not directly in front of them.

35. A: Annular phased array transducers will have crystals that are shaped like discs, which are arranged in a concentric ring to look like a target. The inner active elements will control focusing at shallower depths. Recall that smaller diameter active elements will produce a beam that is focused at a more superficial region.

Deeper focused beams are produced because crystals with a greater diameter allow this. Each ring in an annular phased array will focus at different depths with each becoming deeper than the one before. The end result is an image that comprises only data from each active element's focal zone. A mechanical transducer does fit the criteria for being steered mechanically, but it will have fixed focusing. Linear sequential and convex sequential array transducers allow electronic multifocusing and electronic steering.

36. D: The Fresnel zone is another name for the near zone or near field of the sound wave. This is the region between the transducer and the focal point (which is where the beam is the narrowest). As the sound wave leaves the transducer, it steadily narrows until it reaches the focus. It is at the focal point where the sound beam is half of the diameter of the crystal. The beam is equal to 13 mm at the transducer face.

37. C: The amount of divergence that occurs in the far field (the Fraunhofer zone) is not determined only by the frequency of the soundwave but also by the diameter of the crystal. The diameter of the crystal and the amount of divergence in the far zone are inversely related. For example, a small crystal diameter results in a beam that generates a greater amount of divergence in the far field. Conversely, a larger diameter PZT crystal will result in a beam that is narrower (a lower amount of divergence). Line density and speed do not affect the amount of divergence. The focal zone depth is directly affected by the frequency and the crystal diameter. For example, if a higher frequency is used, there will be a deeper focal depth. Also, a smaller crystal diameter results in a focal depth that is in a shallower location.

38. B: When using a linear sequential array transducer, the image is rectangular. These modern transducers have the capability of being electronically steered and thus would become shaped like a parallelogram instead of a rectangle. The image will never be wider than the probe's footprint. These transducers have a relatively small footprint, and the PZT crystals are located next to each other across the transducer face. These probes have about 120–250 pieces of the active element used to create the sound beam. Linear phased array and annular phased array transducers generate images that are fan or sector shaped. The convex array produces an image that is known as a blunted sector shape.

39. C: Continuous wave (CW) transducer technology uses two active elements. One crystal is constantly sending out sound waves, whereas the other is always on the receiving end. The location of the signals cannot be determined because everything in the path of the sound wave is being recorded, which means there is a lack of range resolution (also referred to as range ambiguity). These transducers are extremely sensitive in picking up Doppler signals (because they do not have backing material), such as fetal heart tones or ankle pulses, but they cannot be used to generate ultrasound images. The other choices in this question are all examples of imaging transducers that do provide images with range resolution.

40. A: To determine if the beam is steered while using a linear phased array transducer, an imaginary line can be drawn connecting the electrical spikes. A straight line indicates that there is no beam steering. If a rise or fall in the line that connects the electrical spikes is noted, steering of the ultrasound beam has taken place. In this image, a definite slope is apparent as the electrical spikes are moving up when passing from left to right. Next, draw a second imaginary line perpendicular to the slope so a T shape is formed. This demonstrates the direction in which the beam will be steered. In this instance, the beam will be steered 45 degrees to the right. This method can be used even if the beam is focused; however, the electrical spikes will not be in a straight line but will take on a curved appearance.

41. D: Focusing is achieved in linear phased array transducers when the electronic spikes are in a curved configuration, known as the electronic curve. If the electronic spikes are not curved, an unfocused wave is created. The electronic slope determines the direction in which the ultrasound wave will be steered. The dynamic aperture is used in array transducers to change the width of the ultrasound wave. PZT crystals are the active elements that create ringing in the transducer when they are excited.

42. B: Range ambiguity is an imaging error in which returning echoes have not yet been returned to the probe before the next pulse is transmitted. If a sonographer increases the imaging depth, the system automatically decreases the pulse repetition frequency (PRF) to avoid range ambiguity. If the PRF is too high while scanning a structure deep in the body, range ambiguity may occur and the system will incorrectly place the received reflections closer to the probe than their actual depth. PRF represents the number of pulses sent into the body every second and is presented in units of hertz (Hz). The PRF is inversely related to the imaging depth, so if the scan depth is twice as deep, the ultrasound system will automatically reduce the PRF by half. The number of scan lines or the persistence is not affected by the imaging depth. The PRP is also determined by the imaging depth, but they have a direct relationship. For example, if the imaging depth is increased, the PRP will also increase. The PRP is the duration from the beginning of one pulse to the next.

43. A: When a sonographer applies focusing during an exam, many changes take place within the ultrasound beam. Near-zone resolution is enhanced. When focusing is used, the energy of the beam is concentrated into one small area (focus), thus improving the lateral resolution. A focused beam also tends to move the focal point closer to the face of the probe being used. This will result in a near-zone length that is shorter when compared to an unfocused beam. Although the ultrasound beam's shape changes, the width is also changed. The beam's diameter will diverge more in the far field, which diminishes the lateral resolution in the far zone.

44. C: If a sonographer scans a blood vessel with B-mode (also referred to as brightness mode), or grayscale, ultrasound, the image will typically appear anechoic because the reflections are not strong enough for visualization. A structure that is anechoic is free from internal echoes. Of course, the ultrasound operator will use color flow Doppler to provide more information pertaining to the blood flow. Hyperechoic involves structures that appear brighter than neighboring tissues. Isogenic describes tissues that display the same amount of brightness on grayscale imaging. Heterogeneous describes a variance of echoes in the tissue that is being evaluated.

45. B: Ultrasound machines are designed to calculate the speed of the ultrasound wave in soft tissue as 1.54mm/μs. The time of flight (go-return time) refers to the time it takes for a pulse to leave the transducer, hit a reflector, and return to the transducer. The depth of the reflector can be calculated as being 1 cm when the time of flight equals 13 μs. Using this rule, if a target is 2 cm deep, the time of flight will be twice as long, equating to 26 μs. If the time of flight takes 39μs, the depth of the reflector will be 3 cm.

46. D: Grayscale imaging requires the use of pulsed wave ultrasound to create an image. Recall that continuous wave (CW) ultrasound, although extremely sensitive, cannot produce an image. Clinically, pulsed wave ultrasound enables the ultrasound system to determine the depth of the reflector by calculating the go-return time, which enables image production. A shorter go-return time correlates with a reflector that is at a shallower depth than one that has a longer go-return time, which is associated with a reflector that is located deeper in the body. Penetration is determined by the output power. Temporal resolution is affected by the imaging depth because a greater depth will result in poorer temporal resolution. The bandwidth refers to the available frequencies in the pulse.

47. C: When the user adjusts the receiver gain on an ultrasound system, it is the amplification that is modified. This action takes place in the receiver, and it has a uniform effect on the image by changing the strength of the voltages that the probe has produced. If the receiver gain is increased, a brighter image will appear throughout the entire image. If the gain is decreased, the overall image becomes darker. Demodulation cannot be adjusted by the user. Reject discards the weak signals. Compression is used to modify the grayscale maps.

48. C: M-mode (also referred to as motion mode) is commonly used during echocardiograms to evaluate heart valve and wall motion as the heart is beating. It is also used to obtain a fetal heart rate during obstetrical ultrasounds. The information that is depicted during M-mode is the amplitude, motion, and time. The user will witness lines moving across the screen when M-mode is employed. Time is represented by the x-axis. The y-axis correlates with the depth of the reflector, and the brightness of the dots corresponds to the amplitude. M-mode displays excellent temporal resolution because only one line is being assessed. Depth and amplitude describe A-mode (also referred to as amplitude mode) with the x-axis representing the depth and the y-axis corresponding to the amplitude. B-mode is grayscale imaging with the depth being determined by the x-axis and amplitude correlating to the z-axis.

49. B: The dynamic range is a ratio of signals that can be portrayed by a system while still containing accurate information. This controls how the intensity of the signals is transformed into shades of gray. This will either increase or limit the different shades of gray. If the image displayed on an ultrasound system has a high amount of contrast, it means that the pixels are either black or white. High-contrast images portray few shades of gray. Therefore, if only black and white are displayed, then there is a narrow dynamic range. A dynamic range that shows many shades of gray would be considered to have a wide dynamic range. These images will be considered to be of low contrast.

50. D: Output gain is one of several names that describes the power of the ultrasound system. Other names for power include output power, output, and acoustic power. The pulser is the component of the ultrasound system that regulates the intensity of the beam that the patient is exposed to. A higher output gain (power) will also increase the ability to scan at greater depths while decreasing the amount of noise present during the scan. Pulse duration and frequency are not related to the output gain used during the exam.

51. A: Tissue harmonics is a technology that is available to correct the malformation of the ultrasound wave that takes place as the sound wave travels into the body. The transmitted, or fundamental, frequency is the frequency of the ultrasound beam that is produced by the transducer and imparted into the patient, and it is responsible for image production. However, during tissue harmonics, this frequency tends to be excluded so that the only signal being used is the harmonic frequency. The harmonic frequency is created within the patient's body and will be two times larger than the fundamental frequency, improving contrast resolution. For example, if the fundamental frequency is 6 MHz, the harmonic frequency will be 12 MHz. An ultrasound beam that is created with harmonic frequencies will not undergo as much distortion and is less likely to produce images with artifacts. When harmonics are used, a strong signal is required, and these signals will be located within the main axis of the sound wave. Spatial compounding can be used to eliminate edge shadows. Overall gain is another name for the process of amplification.

52. B: The gallbladder is an organ that is subject to image artifacts when scanned with ultrasound. It can be difficult to discern if reflectors visualized within it are real. Tissue harmonics is a concept that has helped clinicians and operators gain diagnostic confidence because it tends to eliminate some signals that are not pathological. Harmonic frequencies allow the sonographer to scan patients at higher frequencies that will not only improve the axial resolution but the lateral resolution as well. The lateral resolution tends to improve because the wave is narrower. The use of harmonic frequencies makes it easier to image gallbladders and those organs that are deeper in the body, and it eliminates reverberation artifacts. Reverberation artifacts can mimic sludge within the gallbladder.

53. C: Write zoom can also be referred to as write magnification. This is a type of zoom that can be performed before the image is stored in the scan converter, which makes this a preprocessing function. The spatial resolution is superior because once the image is converted from analog to digital, only the information within the region of interest will be scanned again, creating more pixels and thus resulting in better spatial resolution. Read magnification is a postprocessing function because it can be performed only on an image that has been frozen. This results in pixels that are bigger than the original and will not improve the resolution. Read magnification is also known as read zoom. Temporal resolution can be referred to as the frame rate and may be better if write magnification is used.

54. A: If a sonographer notices that the image is being affected by electronic noise, it may be necessary to adjust the reject on the ultrasound system. The reject function is also referred to as rejection, threshold, or even suppression. Reject is the last process that takes place in the receiver. This function is typically offered in two forms: one that takes place automatically and one that can be controlled by the operator. The reject enables the user to decide if low-level echoes should be displayed within the image, but it does not suppress brighter signals. Sometimes, weaker signals will offer important data for a diagnosis, but clinicians often do not want noise to be present on the image. When the sonographer adjusts the amplification, the whole image will become brighter or darker. Compression allows the user to select the grayscale maps. Demodulation cannot be controlled by the sonographer, and it does not affect the appearance of the ultrasound exam.

55. D: If a sonographer finds it necessary to improve an image while scanning the kidneys (renal ultrasound), it is possible for the operator to adjust the output power, which controls the intensity of the beam. The amplitude can also be modified by increasing or decreasing the amount of receiver gain. The frequency can also be adjusted by increasing or decreasing the frequency that a particular transducer offers or by switching probes. The speed of sound does not depend on any component of the ultrasound machine, but rather the medium, and it cannot be changed by the sonographer. The speed will change only if the type of tissue changes.

56. C: An application that can be used to assist in better visualization of fibroids is coded excitation, which occurs in the pulser. Penetration and resolution are two important factors when considering the quality of an ultrasound image. Higher resolution is obtained using short pulses during an ultrasound exam. Coded excitation allows longer pulses across a variety of frequencies to improve the resolution and allow for deeper penetration, which is often necessary when scanning uterine fibroids. It is possible to apply multiple focal zones with coded excitation. With better penetration and increased resolution in the far field, fibroids are easier to correctly diagnose when using transvaginal transducers. Persistence uses data from images that have already been acquired to improve the quality of the image. Spatial compounding generates an image by acquiring data from angles that can eliminate certain artifacts and can be performed only with phased array technology. Elastography provides information pertaining to the stiffness of the structure being examined.

57. B: If the sharpness of a subtle mass located within the liver needs to be improved, edge enhancement can be applied. This is a technique that allows for better delineation of the border of structures by sharpening the edges of a mass. Edge enhancement sharpens the borders by raising the amount of image contrast at the interface of these tissues. At the boundary between two or more tissue types, shades of gray are displayed, and edge enhancement portrays edges that are more reflective to help the mass stand out more against normal liver tissue that can be identified in the background. Zoom is a technique that is used to magnify an image or part of an image. Fill-in interpolation is a preprocessing technique that provides information about missing data based on what is located between scan lines. If the sonographer increases the receiver gain, this will make the entire image brighter.

58. D: This ultrasound beam has been created with a linear phased array transducer, which is focused and steered to the left. When examining the picture, it is important to note that there is a curvature of the electrical spikes. This curved design governs the focusing of a phased array transducer, which is present. If it were an unfocused beam, the electrical spikes would be in a straight line. Next, it is necessary to determine the direction in which the beam is being steered, which can be done by drawing a straight line and connecting the spikes from left to right. Intersect this line with another that is perpendicular (90 degrees) to discern the direction in which the beam will be steered (in this case, to the left).

59. C: Frequency compounding is an averaging method that tends to take the speckle patterns of multiple images into consideration to reduce the noise and speckle that are produced. Ultrasound images are filled with speckle, but it is important that a reduction takes place to discern objects that demonstrate low contrast. Targets that are smaller may not be visualized if the amount of speckle is not reduced. Spatial compounding can reduce the amount of shadowing and speckle, but instead of averaging multiple frequencies, this method includes data from various angles. Tissue harmonics develop within the patient and are generated within the main ultrasound beam. Temporal compounding is also known as persistence, and although it can be useful to reduce the speckle pattern, it overlaps data from prior frame rates onto the most recent information to smooth out the image.

60. D: The receiver is one of the main components of the ultrasound machine. The receiver is responsible for changing and displaying the signal that is sent from the transducer to the monitor or whichever type of viewing format is being used. This is the fourth component after the transducer, pulser, and beam former, which, as the name suggests, shapes the ultrasound beam. The master synchronizer controls the collaboration of the synergy of the ultrasound components, and storage is the component that is responsible for saving the images and video clips.

61. A: The receiver (also known as the signal processor) has five functions that occur during image production. The receiver obtains the echoes after they have been sent into the patient but before this information is sent to the monitor. Note that these functions are in alphabetical order to help recall them, which puts the series in the following order: amplification, compensation, compression, demodulation, and reject. It should be noted that the modification of the receiver operations does not affect patient exposure because these steps take place when the signal is leaving the patient. Of these functions, demodulation is the only one that cannot be modified with a control on the machine and has no effect on the appearance of the image.

62. B: Preprocessing should be thought of as any change of the image that occurs before the user freezes the image. Examples of preprocessing are adjusting the TGC or gain. Preprocessing occurs before the data are sent to the scan converter to be stored. The scan converter is responsible for taking a number and converting the information to grayscale. The pulser determines the intensity of the ultrasound beam. The receiver receives the signal from the patient and prepares it for image display. The beam former works with phased array transducers and determines how the ultrasound beam will be steered and focused.

63. C: Persistence (also called temporal averaging or temporal compounding) is a method that can be used during grayscale or color Doppler imaging. It can be adjusted by the user. By overlapping information obtained from older frames onto more recent images obtained, the machine can produce an ultrasound image with greater detail that has less noise, is smoother, and has an improved signal-to-noise ratio. If the signal-to-noise ratio is higher than the useless low-level echoes, the system will get rid of the noise. Less noise is desired during image production. Although the image detail improves with the use of temporal compounding, temporal resolution is degraded because of the additional processing. This makes imaging structures that are moving rapidly difficult to image because there will be a lag as temporal resolution is decreased. Persistence is best used with structures that demonstrate slow motion, such as slow blood flow.

64. B: Voxel stands for volume element, and it is the smallest element of a picture that has been generated with 3D technology. The difference between a voxel and a pixel is that the latter refers to a 2D image. Pixels are the tiny boxes that will each have their own gray shade to make up a digital image. To produce an image with greater resolution, a higher pixel density is required. Pixel density is the number of boxes per inch on the display. A high pixel density will offer better resolution because there will be more pixels found in every inch of the image. A bit has a value equal to either 1 or 0, and it refers to the smallest unit of data that a computer can store. Bit is the abbreviation for binary digit. In computer language, there are 8 bits in 1 byte.

65. D: The Digital Imaging and Communications in Medicine (DICOM) system is the necessary link between the ultrasound machine (or any other digital imaging system) and the picture archiving and communications system (PACS), the component responsible for archiving and transferring images. DICOM allows for the integration of a facility's networks, printing devices, workstations, and PACS system. The DICOM protocols allow the ultrasound machine to send the images to the PACS network for archiving purposes. In contrast to JPEG images, DICOM images are extremely large, and they cannot be loaded onto regular computers. A DICOM browser is necessary so that the images can be viewed on computers, workstations, or even a CD. A bit is the smallest unit of information in computer language. RIS is an acronym for radiology information system, which is an electronic health record specific to radiology departments for scheduling, tracking patients, and billing functions.

66. B: PACS allows users of digital imaging equipment to electronically share and archive images. This is an important tool that gives clinicians and other medical personnel access to images as well reports that have been generated. PACS has been used to replace film for facilities that have converted to digital imaging systems. This not only saves storage space for film and chemicals used to process film within departments, but it also allows more than one user to visualize studies at the same time as well as it grants instantaneous access to the stored images. Over time, film studies tend to deteriorate; this will not occur with studies that are archived with a PACS system. RIS is an electronic health record specific to radiology departments for scheduling, tracking patients, and billing functions. A bit is the smallest unit of information in computer language. DICOM is a necessary link between the ultrasound machine (or any other digital imaging system) and the PACS system, and it allows for the integration of the facility's networks, printing devices, workstations, and PACS system.

67. D: The progression of the signal through an ultrasound machine is first the transducer, which contains the PZT crystal. Next is the receiver, which will change the probe's electrical signal so that it can eventually be visualized on the monitor. The scan converter is responsible for changing the data from analog to digital, and digital to analog, as well as controlling the system's memory. The display is the component that allows the operator to view the images generated by the system.

68. A: A pixel is the smallest portion of a 2D image that is in a digital format. Pixel density refers to the number of pixels contained in every inch of the image. The more pixels that an image contains, the better the spatial resolution. A high pixel density will dramatically improve an image, whether it is on a digital camera, flat-screen TV, or ultrasound display. In this example, analog and digital display are added as additional information to throw the reader off, but if better spatial resolution is desired, the user must choose the $1,500 \times 1,500$ analog display because of the higher pixel count that generates 2,250,000 pixels (multiply $1,500 \times 1,500$).

69. C: If the radiologist requests an image with as much anatomy as possible, the sonographer could use the extended field of view (EFOV) control on the ultrasound system. This application can be used when interrogating a Baker's cyst, the length of the Achilles tendon, or the abdominal aorta to provide additional information regarding the exact location of aneurysms or other pathology that may be encountered. This panoramic image is available on most modern ultrasound equipment and replaces the split-screen method of demonstrating objects that are longer than the transducer face. By acquiring volume data, the system will stitch the information together to display one image. Often, anatomical structures are enlarged, and it may be difficult to obtain measurements. Other uses include exams of the thyroid, testes, or breast lesions, and musculoskeletal exams, . Elastography is an application that measures tissue stiffness. Color Doppler will typically be used during evaluation of the abdominal aorta, but this application provides information related to the Doppler shift of the blood flow. B-mode is grayscale imaging, which is used to generate ultrasound images, but EFOV is the choice that will allow the greatest field of view.

70. A: The horizontal axis of a TGC curve refers to how much compensation is necessary for the depth of the object being imaged (vertical axis). The top of the vertical axis represents the patient's skin, and as it moves down, it refers to tissues that are located deeper in the body. The near gain is located superficially near the skin's surface. At this location, the structures being imaged need little TGC because not much attenuation occurs. The slope is the middle portion of the TGC curve in which more compensation is necessary because of the greater depths. The knee is located at the distal portion of the slope, and it demonstrates where the most compensation will occur. The region of the far gain is distal to the knee and even deeper, which designates the greatest amount of compensation offered by the machine. Phase quadrature is not a component of the TGC curve.

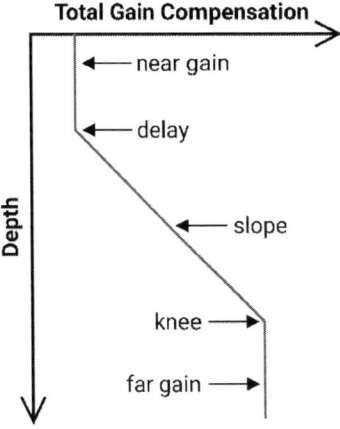

71. B: A bit has a value equal to either 1 or 0, and it is the smallest unit of data that a computer can store. To calculate the number of shades of gray in 3 bits of memory, one would take 2 to the nth power, with n equal to the number of bits. In this instance, $2^3 = 2 \times 2 \times 2 = 8$. This demonstrates that in 3 bits of memory, one can see eight different shades of gray.

72. D: Contrast resolution can be thought of as the ability to see the differences in intensities in tissues that are beside each other on a grayscale image. Ultrasound images that contain many shades of gray will offer better contrast resolution. To calculate the number of shades of gray in a specific number of bits of memory, one would take 2 to the nth power, with n equal to the number of bits. Four bits is equal to 2 to the 4th power ($2 \times 2 \times 2 \times 2$), which is equal to 16 different shades of gray. Two hundred fifty-six shades of gray would be 2 to the 8th power, which is equal to

8 bits. Thirty-two shades of gray would be 2 to the 5th power, which is 5 bits. Sixteen bits is equal to 65,536 shades of gray, so, of the options listed, this will offer the highest amount of gray shades and provide the best contrast resolution.

73. D: During a carotid duplex exam, if a sonographer is using pulsed wave Doppler to determine the peak velocity of blood flow in a carotid artery, the operator must remember that when the red blood cells are moving along the same path of the ultrasound beam, the most accurate measurements will be obtained. Thus, the Doppler shift (otherwise known as the Doppler frequency) will be highest at 0 (flow moving toward the transducer) or 180 degrees (flow moving away from the transducer). If the angle between the target and reflector is anything other than 0 or 180 degrees, the velocity is less precise. If an operator tries to interrogate a structure at a 90-degree angle with pulsed wave Doppler, no Doppler shift will take place because the frequency shift cannot be identified because the cosine of 90 degrees is equal to 0.

74. C: When an ultrasound operator wants to measure velocities within a blood vessel, pulsed wave Doppler can be used. The advantage of pulsed wave (over CW) Doppler is that the sonographer can place the gate (sample volume) in a location of choice to obtain the best measurements. The gate should be placed in the center of the blood vessel.

75. C: This is a spectral Doppler waveform of the patient's left internal carotid artery (ICA) that indicates a significant amount of plaque in the proximal portion of the left ICA. This spectral waveform of the mid-left ICA displays a peak systolic velocity (PSV) of 479.6 cm/s, with an end-diastolic velocity (EDV) of 151.7 cm/s. Because the PSV is greater than 125 cm/s and the EDV is more than 140 cm/s, it is estimated that the diameter reduction of the left ICA is 80–99%. The Doppler signal was obtained with the angle correction of 60 degrees, and the sample volume was placed distal to the stenosis. The waveform also demonstrates a considerable amount of spectral broadening.

76. B: The pressure within the venous system is influenced by a patient's breathing patterns due to the fact that it is a low-pressure system and due to the movement of the diaphragm with inspiration and expiration. If a sonographer asks the patient to take in a deep breath and hold it, this is referred to as inhalation, or inspiration. With inspiration, venous flow rate in the legs decreases because the diaphragm descends into the abdominal cavity. This downward movement of the diaphragm increases pressure within the abdominal cavity. Conversely, upon expiration, the diaphragm ascends into the chest cavity, which decreases venous blood flow from above the level of the heart while increasing the amount of pressure in the chest. Turbulent flow is often present distal to a stenosis. Pulsatile flow is associated with the contraction of the heart and is typically present when evaluating the arterial system with Doppler.

77. A: Sonographers should immediately identify these images as typical blood flow patterns in which the red blood cells are moving through the vessel when no pathology is present. Laminar flow is the type of flow that is exhibited in normal anatomical structures. This flow is layered and smooth and travels parallel along the length of the vessel. There are two configurations regarding laminar flow. The first picture represents a parabolic pattern that tends to have velocities that are higher in the middle of the vessel with slower velocity flow along the walls. The shape that is created with a parabolic flow pattern is like a bullet. The second image demonstrates plug flow, which will have the same velocity in all of the layers present. A blood vessel that contains laminar flow will produce a Reynolds number of less than 1,500. The Reynolds number is a way to forecast if the flow will be laminar or turbulent. Turbulent flow will have a Reynolds number that is greater than 2,000. Turbulent flow is also associated with chaotic blood flow and eddy currents.

78. A: The 14 MHz transducer will display a Doppler shift that is greater than that of the 7 MHz transducer. Higher frequency transducers generate greater Doppler shifts, and there is a direct relationship between the Doppler shift and transducer frequency. In this instance, the Doppler shift was doubled when switching from a 7 MHz to a 14 MHz transducer. If the sonographer would have started with a 14 MHz transducer and then used the 7 MHz probe, the Doppler shift would have been halved.

79. C: The error that is depicted in this image is known as aliasing. Aliasing is a common artifact witnessed in color Doppler and in spectral Doppler. There are many steps that can be taken to eliminate signals that display aliasing. The first step a sonographer should try is to adjust the pulse repetition frequency (PRF), which is also known as the velocity scale. Because this is an artery, the blood flow is moving rapidly, so increasing the PRF may help unwrap the spectral display. This step increases the Nyquist limit, which is also known as the aliasing frequency and is equal to half of the PRF. If this alone does not take care of aliasing, the baseline may be adjusted accordingly. In this situation, dropping the baseline down closer to the bottom of the window will help alleviate the appearance of aliasing. Another helpful tip to eliminate aliasing is to switch to a lower frequency transducer or even to find a window that is at a shallower location. The sonographer could also use continuous wave (CW) Doppler because aliasing will never occur, since aliasing is exclusively inherent with pulsed Doppler.

80. A: Pulsed wave Doppler is a useful method to measure blood flow velocities within blood vessels. The user has the option to select where the gate should be placed within a vessel to take a velocity measurement and know the exact location of this reading. However, sometimes the velocity within the blood vessel is too high, and the operator is unable to obtain a peak velocity measurement that is accurate. The sonographer would want to switch to continuous wave (CW) Doppler because velocities that are extremely high tend to be more accurate because there will not be a maximum velocity while using this method. While using pulsed wave Doppler, if the user cannot eliminate aliasing after changing the scale or depth of the target or switching to a lower frequency probe, one will be successful if switching to CW Doppler.

81. D: The aliasing frequency is also referred to as the Nyquist limit. This number can be calculated by dividing the pulse repetition frequency (PRF) by 2. Aliasing will be apparent if the Doppler frequency is higher than the Nyquist limit. Therefore, to prevent aliasing, the sonographer will want to raise the Nyquist limit. This can be done by raising the PRF scale: If the PRF is increased, so is the Nyquist limit. One may also raise the Nyquist limit by finding a new sonographic window that is at a shallower location. The PRF is controlled by the reflector depth. If the target is deeper in the body, the PRF will be low, as will the Nyquist limit. This decreased value makes the ultrasound system more susceptible to aliasing. When we divide the PRF (which is 8) by 2, it equals 4 kHz.

82. C: Color Doppler is a pulsed wave technique that demonstrates a Doppler frequency shift that overlays a grayscale image with the use of autocorrelation. Color Doppler is a pulsed wave technique; therefore, aliasing may occur. Due to it being a pulsed wave method, range resolution does exist when using color Doppler. Color Doppler is not used to measure the peak systolic and end diastolic velocities but rather the mean velocity and direction of a moving target.

83. B: PRF stands for pulse repetition frequency but is also referred to as the scale while pulsed Doppler is being used. In this example, the vessel being interrogated displays blood flow that is moving slowly. If color is not optimized after turning on color Doppler, the sonographer would want to decrease the PRF so that the ultrasound system is more receptive in picking up slower blood flow signals. Blood that is within the venous portion of the circulatory system is often blood that moves more slowly. If this step alone does not improve the color Doppler visualization of the vessel, the sonographer may need to increase the color gain. If the operator chose to increase the PRF scale, a decreased sensitivity to slow flow will be noted. However, if one is interrogating a vessel with higher velocity flow, the PRF should be set higher to raise the Nyquist limit and prevent or eliminate aliasing. Adjusting the PRF does affect the visualization of blood flow, which makes incorrect.

84. A: In general, a Doppler shift is produced when an ultrasound wave collides with a red blood cell that is in motion, which means that a Doppler shift is absolutely present. It must be determined, however, if the shift will be positive or negative. If the red blood cells are traveling in a direction that is in the opposite direction of the transducer, a negative Doppler shift would take place. When the red blood cells are moving in the direction of the transducer, the result is a frequency that is reflected and is greater than the frequency of the transmitted signal. This demonstrates a positive Doppler shift (also known as the Doppler frequency). The amount of Doppler shift that occurs is directly proportional to the frequency of the transducer. Therefore, if an exam is repeated with a transducer that has a frequency that is twice as high as what was used in the first exam, the Doppler shift (frequency) will be doubled. Unequivocal is not a viable option for this question.

85. C: Aliasing occurs when the spectral waveform tends to wind around the spectral window. Carotid duplex exams are performed with linear sequential transducers. Aliasing will be eliminated when a lower frequency transducer is being used, and, in this example, if the sonographer started with 10 MHz, the next step would be to switch to the 7 MHz linear sequential transducer. A 4.5 MHz curved array transducer, although a lower frequency, is not a transducer that is used to complete carotid exams. Higher frequency probes are more prone to aliasing artifacts because the Doppler shift is calculated using the frequency of the transducer and, in turn, it has a direct relationship. Doppler shifts will be smaller when lower frequency probes are used, so aliasing does not occur as often with lower frequency transducers.

86. B: When a sonographer is using routine grayscale ultrasound imaging, it has been proven that the ideal incident beam is when the transducer is placed 90 degrees to the object being scanned. By using the Doppler equation, however, the cosine of 90 degrees is equal to 0. This indicates that the ultrasound system will not pick up a Doppler frequency when the angle of incidence is 90 degrees (perpendicular) to the direction of blood flow and needs to be changed. If the sonographer saw the movement of blood cells on grayscale imaging, this is a great clue that the blood vessel is not obstructed. Although using power Doppler is an option, it is important to try to optimize color Doppler first because power Doppler does not provide information pertaining to the direction or speed of blood flow. Calling maintenance is likely not necessary unless several attempts of modifying the angle of incidence, increasing the color gain, and adjusting the scale fail to demonstrate color. If this is still the case, one may conclude that the color Doppler is not working correctly and maintenance should be called.

87. A: If a sonographer notices that the lower velocities are missing from the spectral waveform, the wall filter control can be decreased so that the lower frequency shifts appear along the baseline. It is important to note that the wall filter does not affect blood flow that is moving at a higher velocity and tends to get rid of the shifts that are the result of anatomical motion. The scale is the pulse repetition frequency (PRF), and this can be adjusted if the spectral waveform is aliasing. If aliasing occurs, the scale should be increased. Changing the depth will not help demonstrate the lower frequency velocities. The gain of the spectral Doppler waveform can be increased or decreased, but this will affect only the appearance of the grayscale data within the spectral window and is used to eliminate any noise that may be evident.

88. D: The Reynolds number is a value that predicts the flow patterns of blood; it is a unitless number that be calculated from the following equation:

$$\text{Reynolds number} = \frac{(\text{average flow speed}) \times (\text{vessel diameter}) \times (\text{density})}{(\text{viscosity})}$$

If the calculated value is less than 1,500, laminar flow will be present. It should be noted that plug flow is a type of laminar flow. Disturbed flow will fall between 1,500 and 2,000. If the value is more than 2,000 it is predicted that turbulent flow will be visualized, and in this instance, the flow is predicted to be turbulent because it is 2,078. As seen with the equation, if there is increased speed of flow, there will be a higher Reynolds number. If the diameter of the vessel is larger, the Reynolds number will also be greater. Density has the same effect on this calculation. The Reynolds number has an indirect relationship with the viscosity of the blood.

89. C: During a carotid duplex exam, if color appears to be bleeding outside of the artery when color Doppler is applied, it is known as a ghosting artifact. Ghosting and clutter are both low-frequency Doppler shifts that initiate artifacts from anatomical motion, such as the arterial wall. Clutter is associated with the spectral waveform, and when this low-frequency shift is seen with color Doppler, it is referred to as ghosting. Crosstalk is seen on a spectral display only when blood flow appears bidirectional when it truly is unidirectional. Pulsed Doppler can create aliasing, which is the most prevalent artifact when color or spectral Doppler is used.

90. A: Spectral analysis with pulsed wave Doppler allows users to see, hear, and measure blood flow velocities. The spectral window is the clear, black region between the baseline and the spectral line. When this area is filled in and there is widening of the line, spectral broadening is indicated. Spectral broadening is typical when turbulent (high-velocity) blood flow is sampled. This turbulence comprises many areas of flow reversal and velocities, and flow may be seen beneath the baseline. If the ICA is being interrogated and the sonographer can visualize a tight stenosis, one would not be surprised to see spectral broadening. Instead of a clear spectral window, which is expected in a patent ICA or laminar flow, it appears to be filled in, which represents spectral broadening. If the gain is set too high, noise will be apparent throughout the entire window.

91. B: Sometimes, the sonographer will notice that blood flow from arteries and veins is being displayed. Modern systems will have a triplex function that allows the user to display grayscale, color Doppler, and spectral Doppler at the same time. If the user is picking up flow from two different vessels, they should update the triplex image, and move the sample volume into the vessel of interest. Angle correction is necessary to measure the velocities of the blood within a vessel. The sweep speed controls the number of seconds that are shown at once. Pulse repetition frequency (PRF) is the scale that represents the pulses generated every second by the system.

92. D: Color Doppler will allow velocity information to be portrayed as an overlay of color on the traditional grayscale image. To optimize temporal resolution, the user needs to be aware of the size and location of the color box. As the color box size increases, the frame rate, or temporal resolution, decreases because more information needs to be processed. This is especially important when considering the width of the color box. More scan lines are required with a wider color box, and more time is required by the system to process the acquired data. The sonographer should limit the size of the color box to the anatomy of interest and most importantly decrease the width of the color box. The location is also something to consider because a deeper location may be prone to aliasing of the color flow because the pulse repetition frequency (PRF) is lower. The angle of the color box and gain will not affect temporal resolution.

93. B: During a Doppler exam, the only choice that will increase the amount of exposure for the patient in this instance is if the sonographer increases the pulse repetition frequency (PRF). PRF is a control that sonographers are familiar with when using color and pulsed wave Doppler imaging. PRF controls how rapidly data sampling takes place and will allow the ultrasound system to increase or decrease the Doppler shifts that are displayed. A high PRF setting enables more sampling to take place because there is less listening time between the pulses, which equates to more pulses transmitted into the body. It is important to have the PRF set correctly during both modalities so that aliasing does not occur. Color Doppler enables ultrasound users to determine the direction of flow when present and requires eight pulses/scan line. Spectral analysis allows operators to measure velocities as well as provides information about the direction and presence of flow but requires more effort at 256 pulses/scan line. Increasing the Doppler angle, repositioning the baseline to a higher location, and increasing the Doppler gain will not affect the amount of exposure to the patient.

94. C: Pulse repetition frequency (PRF) is the number of pulses sent in one second. When color Doppler is used, many pulses are used for each scan line to increase the sensitivity to low flow and to get a more precise measurement of the velocities. In this instance, the sonographer would want to decrease the packet size to improve the frame rate because less time is required with a smaller packet size. The packet size is also referred to as the ensemble length. An increased packet size tends to degrade temporal resolution because more pulses are being sent out at the same time, which requires more time for data acquisition. Changing the color map and adjusting the color Doppler gain will not affect the frame rate.

95. A: Power Doppler (also referred to as energy mode or color angio) is a form of color Doppler that does not display the speed of blood flow or any directional information. Hence, power Doppler does not evaluate the velocity of the blood flow. Rather, it determines only that a Doppler shift has taken place and shows the amplitude of the moving blood. If there are more red blood cells in one area, the signals will be brighter. Vessels represented with power Doppler will all be identical colors on the display. Advantages of power Doppler include the fact that aliasing does not occur because the speed and direction (velocity) of the blood flow are not applicable. Power Doppler picks up blood flow in smaller vessels and slow blood flow because of its increase in sensitivity. There is an increase in sensitivity because power Doppler is not altered by the Doppler angle.

96. D: Ultrasound operators have several options to eliminate signals that display aliasing. The first step a sonographer should try is to adjust the pulse repetition frequency (PRF,). In this instance, blood is moving through the femoral artery rapidly, so increasing the PRF may help to unwrap the spectral display. This step increases the Nyquist limit, which is also known as the aliasing frequency and is equal to half of the PRF. If this alone does not take care of aliasing, the baseline may be adjusted accordingly. Another helpful tip to eliminate aliasing is to switch to a lower frequency transducer or even find a window that is at a shallower location. The angle of incidence could also be increased to help eliminate aliasing.

97. B: Aliasing can occur with not only spectral Doppler analysis but with color flow Doppler as well. Sonographers must be able to discern between aliasing and the reversal of flow (bidirectional flow). To determine if aliasing is present in the carotid artery, the user must pay close attention to the color map located on the side of the image. If the colors on the map tend to wrap from the top around the outside and to the bottom of the map, then users may assume that aliasing is present. If the colors on the middle of the color map communicate with each other, as stated in this example, then bidirectional flow is present. The wall filter affects only slow flow, which would not affect the blood moving within the carotid artery.

98. B: Color Doppler in a sector-shaped image cannot be steered like it can with a linear transducer. Only the size and location of the color box can be adjusted. Steering of the color box in this instance cannot be performed as it could if a linear transducer were in use. The shape of the color box cannot be changed as it may with a linear transducer when it changes from a rectangle to a parallelogram when steering is employed. The velocities of the moving red blood cells can be determined.

99. A: In this image, note that the color box is almost perpendicular to the blood vessel (but it is not quite 90 degrees, which is why some flow is visible within the lumen while not being completely filled in). The cosine of 90 degrees is equal to 0, which means that no Doppler shift can be detected. Color Doppler works best when the angle between the ultrasound beam and the blood flow is something other than 90 degrees and will enable the machine to display color flow in the blood vessels that are being interrogated. One of the first steps that a sonographer would take in this instance is to change the steering of the color box. It is already steered to the right, but the direction should be changed, and because the vessel is slanted, it should be steered to the left. Another check that a sonographer can do after adjusting the steering is to increase the color gain, which is the opposite of what states. Increasing the output power will not help the color fill of this vessel. Sometimes finding a window that is shallower will help color Doppler, but it is not typically the first step to improve flow.

100. C: Spectral analysis with pulsed wave Doppler allows users to see, hear, and measure blood flow velocities. The spectral window is the clear, black region between the baseline and the spectral line. When this area is filled in and there is widening of the line, spectral broadening is indicated. Spectral broadening is typical when turbulent (high-velocity) blood flow is sampled. This turbulence comprises many areas of flow reversal and velocities, and flow may be seen beneath the baseline. If a velocity measurement is taken within a tight stenosis of the ICA, one would not be surprised to see spectral broadening. This may also be present when small vessels are being investigated or if a velocity is measured distal to a tight stenosis of the ECA. If a sample is obtained in which a vessel bifurcates, it would not be surprising to see spectral broadening. A patent blood vessel is one that is not obstructed, and this is not an instance of when the ultrasound operator would expect to see spectral broadening.

Image Credits

LICENSED UNDER CC BY 4.0 (CREATIVECOMMONS.ORG/LICENSES/BY/4.0/)

Extended Field of View: "panoramic view of an obstructive FLUTD" by Wikimedia user Kalumet (https://commons.wikimedia.org/wiki/File:FLUTD_Sono_Panoramic_view.jpg)

LICENSED UNDER CC BY-SA 3.0 (CREATIVECOMMONS.ORG/LICENSES/BY-SA/3.0/)

Gallstones: "Gallstones" by James Heilman, MD (https://commons.wikimedia.org/wiki/File:Gallstones.PNG)

Stenosis: "Internal carotid artery stenosis" by Wikimedia user Mme Mim (https://commons.wikimedia.org/wiki/File:Internal_carotid_artery_stenosis_in_ultrasound_near_occlusion.jpg)

How to Overcome Test Anxiety

Just the thought of taking a test is enough to make most people a little nervous. A test is an important event that can have a long-term impact on your future, so it's important to take it seriously and it's natural to feel anxious about performing well. But just because anxiety is normal, that doesn't mean that it's helpful in test taking, or that you should simply accept it as part of your life. Anxiety can have a variety of effects. These effects can be mild, like making you feel slightly nervous, or severe, like blocking your ability to focus or remember even a simple detail.

If you experience test anxiety—whether severe or mild—it's important to know how to beat it. To discover this, first you need to understand what causes test anxiety.

Causes of Test Anxiety

While we often think of anxiety as an uncontrollable emotional state, it can actually be caused by simple, practical things. One of the most common causes of test anxiety is that a person does not feel adequately prepared for their test. This feeling can be the result of many different issues such as poor study habits or lack of organization, but the most common culprit is time management. Starting to study too late, failing to organize your study time to cover all of the material, or being distracted while you study will mean that you're not well prepared for the test. This may lead to cramming the night before, which will cause you to be physically and mentally exhausted for the test. Poor time management also contributes to feelings of stress, fear, and hopelessness as you realize you are not well prepared but don't know what to do about it.

Other times, test anxiety is not related to your preparation for the test but comes from unresolved fear. This may be a past failure on a test, or poor performance on tests in general. It may come from comparing yourself to others who seem to be performing better or from the stress of living up to expectations. Anxiety may be driven by fears of the future—how failure on this test would affect your educational and career goals. These fears are often completely irrational, but they can still negatively impact your test performance.

Elements of Test Anxiety

As mentioned earlier, test anxiety is considered to be an emotional state, but it has physical and mental components as well. Sometimes you may not even realize that you are suffering from test anxiety until you notice the physical symptoms. These can include trembling hands, rapid heartbeat, sweating, nausea, and tense muscles. Extreme anxiety may lead to fainting or vomiting. Obviously, any of these symptoms can have a negative impact on testing. It is important to recognize them as soon as they begin to occur so that you can address the problem before it damages your performance.

The mental components of test anxiety include trouble focusing and inability to remember learned information. During a test, your mind is on high alert, which can help you recall information and stay focused for an extended period of time. However, anxiety interferes with your mind's natural processes, causing you to blank out, even on the questions you know well. The strain of testing during anxiety makes it difficult to stay focused, especially on a test that may take several hours. Extreme anxiety can take a huge mental toll, making it difficult not only to recall test information but even to understand the test questions or pull your thoughts together.

Effects of Test Anxiety

Test anxiety is like a disease—if left untreated, it will get progressively worse. Anxiety leads to poor performance, and this reinforces the feelings of fear and failure, which in turn lead to poor performances on subsequent tests. It can grow from a mild nervousness to a crippling condition. If allowed to progress, test anxiety can have a big impact on your schooling, and consequently on your future.

Test anxiety can spread to other parts of your life. Anxiety on tests can become anxiety in any stressful situation, and blanking on a test can turn into panicking in a job situation. But fortunately, you don't have to let anxiety rule your testing and determine your grades. There are a number of relatively simple steps you can take to move past anxiety and function normally on a test and in the rest of life.

Physical Steps for Beating Test Anxiety

While test anxiety is a serious problem, the good news is that it can be overcome. It doesn't have to control your ability to think and remember information. While it may take time, you can begin taking steps today to beat anxiety.

Just as your first hint that you may be struggling with anxiety comes from the physical symptoms, the first step to treating it is also physical. Rest is crucial for having a clear, strong mind. If you are tired, it is much easier to give in to anxiety. But if you establish good sleep habits, your body and mind will be ready to perform optimally, without the strain of exhaustion. Additionally, sleeping well helps you to retain information better, so you're more likely to recall the answers when you see the test questions.

Getting good sleep means more than going to bed on time. It's important to allow your brain time to relax. Take study breaks from time to time so it doesn't get overworked, and don't study right before bed. Take time to rest your mind before trying to rest your body, or you may find it difficult to fall asleep.

Along with sleep, other aspects of physical health are important in preparing for a test. Good nutrition is vital for good brain function. Sugary foods and drinks may give a burst of energy but this burst is followed by a crash, both physically and emotionally. Instead, fuel your body with protein and vitamin-rich foods.

Also, drink plenty of water. Dehydration can lead to headaches and exhaustion, especially if your brain is already under stress from the rigors of the test. Particularly if your test is a long one, drink water during the breaks. And if possible, take an energy-boosting snack to eat between sections.

Along with sleep and diet, a third important part of physical health is exercise. Maintaining a steady workout schedule is helpful, but even taking 5-minute study breaks to walk can help get your blood pumping faster and clear your head. Exercise also releases endorphins, which contribute to a positive feeling and can help combat test anxiety.

When you nurture your physical health, you are also contributing to your mental health. If your body is healthy, your mind is much more likely to be healthy as well. So take time to rest, nourish your body with healthy food and water, and get moving as much as possible. Taking these physical steps will make you stronger and more able to take the mental steps necessary to overcome test anxiety.

Mental Steps for Beating Test Anxiety

Working on the mental side of test anxiety can be more challenging, but as with the physical side, there are clear steps you can take to overcome it. As mentioned earlier, test anxiety often stems from lack of preparation, so the obvious solution is to prepare for the test. Effective studying may be the most important weapon you have for beating test anxiety, but you can and should employ several other mental tools to combat fear.

First, boost your confidence by reminding yourself of past success—tests or projects that you aced. If you're putting as much effort into preparing for this test as you did for those, there's no reason you should expect to fail here. Work hard to prepare; then trust your preparation.

Second, surround yourself with encouraging people. It can be helpful to find a study group, but be sure that the people you're around will encourage a positive attitude. If you spend time with others who are anxious or cynical, this will only contribute to your own anxiety. Look for others who are motivated to study hard from a desire to succeed, not from a fear of failure.

Third, reward yourself. A test is physically and mentally tiring, even without anxiety, and it can be helpful to have something to look forward to. Plan an activity following the test, regardless of the outcome, such as going to a movie or getting ice cream.

When you are taking the test, if you find yourself beginning to feel anxious, remind yourself that you know the material. Visualize successfully completing the test. Then take a few deep, relaxing breaths and return to it. Work through the questions carefully but with confidence, knowing that you are capable of succeeding.

Developing a healthy mental approach to test taking will also aid in other areas of life. Test anxiety affects more than just the actual test—it can be damaging to your mental health and even contribute to depression. It's important to beat test anxiety before it becomes a problem for more than testing.

Study Strategy

Being prepared for the test is necessary to combat anxiety, but what does being prepared look like? You may study for hours on end and still not feel prepared. What you need is a strategy for test prep. The next few pages outline our recommended steps to help you plan out and conquer the challenge of preparation.

STEP 1: SCOPE OUT THE TEST

Learn everything you can about the format (multiple choice, essay, etc.) and what will be on the test. Gather any study materials, course outlines, or sample exams that may be available. Not only will this help you to prepare, but knowing what to expect can help to alleviate test anxiety.

STEP 2: MAP OUT THE MATERIAL

Look through the textbook or study guide and make note of how many chapters or sections it has. Then divide these over the time you have. For example, if a book has 15 chapters and you have five days to study, you need to cover three chapters each day. Even better, if you have the time, leave an extra day at the end for overall review after you have gone through the material in depth.

If time is limited, you may need to prioritize the material. Look through it and make note of which sections you think you already have a good grasp on, and which need review. While you are studying, skim quickly through the familiar sections and take more time on the challenging parts. Write out your plan so you don't get lost as you go. Having a written plan also helps you feel more in control of the study, so anxiety is less likely to arise from feeling overwhelmed at the amount to cover.

STEP 3: GATHER YOUR TOOLS

Decide what study method works best for you. Do you prefer to highlight in the book as you study and then go back over the highlighted portions? Or do you type out notes of the important information? Or is it helpful to make flashcards that you can carry with you? Assemble the pens, index cards, highlighters, post-it notes, and any other materials you may need so you won't be distracted by getting up to find things while you study.

If you're having a hard time retaining the information or organizing your notes, experiment with different methods. For example, try color-coding by subject with colored pens, highlighters, or post-it notes. If you learn better by hearing, try recording yourself reading your notes so you can listen while in the car, working out, or simply sitting at your desk. Ask a friend to quiz you from your flashcards, or try teaching someone the material to solidify it in your mind.

STEP 4: CREATE YOUR ENVIRONMENT

It's important to avoid distractions while you study. This includes both the obvious distractions like visitors and the subtle distractions like an uncomfortable chair (or a too-comfortable couch that makes you want to fall asleep). Set up the best study environment possible: good lighting and a comfortable work area. If background music helps you focus, you may want to turn it on, but otherwise keep the room quiet. If you are using a computer to take notes, be sure you don't have any other windows open, especially applications like social media, games, or anything else that could distract you. Silence your phone and turn off notifications. Be sure to keep water close by so you stay hydrated while you study (but avoid unhealthy drinks and snacks).

Also, take into account the best time of day to study. Are you freshest first thing in the morning? Try to set aside some time then to work through the material. Is your mind clearer in the afternoon or evening? Schedule your study session then. Another method is to study at the same time of day that you will take the test, so that your brain gets used to working on the material at that time and will be ready to focus at test time.

STEP 5: STUDY!

Once you have done all the study preparation, it's time to settle into the actual studying. Sit down, take a few moments to settle your mind so you can focus, and begin to follow your study plan. Don't give in to distractions or let yourself procrastinate. This is your time to prepare so you'll be ready to fearlessly approach the test. Make the most of the time and stay focused.

Of course, you don't want to burn out. If you study too long you may find that you're not retaining the information very well. Take regular study breaks. For example, taking five minutes out of every hour to walk briskly, breathing deeply and swinging your arms, can help your mind stay fresh.

As you get to the end of each chapter or section, it's a good idea to do a quick review. Remind yourself of what you learned and work on any difficult parts. When you feel that you've mastered the material, move on to the next part. At the end of your study session, briefly skim through your notes again.

But while review is helpful, cramming last minute is NOT. If at all possible, work ahead so that you won't need to fit all your study into the last day. Cramming overloads your brain with more information than it can process and retain, and your tired mind may struggle to recall even previously learned information when it is overwhelmed with last-minute study. Also, the urgent nature of cramming and the stress placed on your brain contribute to anxiety. You'll be more likely to go to the test feeling unprepared and having trouble thinking clearly.

So don't cram, and don't stay up late before the test, even just to review your notes at a leisurely pace. Your brain needs rest more than it needs to go over the information again. In fact, plan to finish your studies by noon or early afternoon the day before the test. Give your brain the rest of the day to relax or focus on other things, and get a good night's sleep. Then you will be fresh for the test and better able to recall what you've studied.

STEP 6: TAKE A PRACTICE TEST

Many courses offer sample tests, either online or in the study materials. This is an excellent resource to check whether you have mastered the material, as well as to prepare for the test format and environment.

Check the test format ahead of time: the number of questions, the type (multiple choice, free response, etc.), and the time limit. Then create a plan for working through them. For example, if you have 30 minutes to take a 60-question test, your limit is 30 seconds per question. Spend less time on the questions you know well so that you can take more time on the difficult ones.

If you have time to take several practice tests, take the first one open book, with no time limit. Work through the questions at your own pace and make sure you fully understand them. Gradually work up to taking a test under test conditions: sit at a desk with all study materials put away and set a timer. Pace yourself to make sure you finish the test with time to spare and go back to check your answers if you have time.

After each test, check your answers. On the questions you missed, be sure you understand why you missed them. Did you misread the question (tests can use tricky wording)? Did you forget the information? Or was it something you hadn't learned? Go back and study any shaky areas that the practice tests reveal.

Taking these tests not only helps with your grade, but also aids in combating test anxiety. If you're already used to the test conditions, you're less likely to worry about it, and working through tests until you're scoring well gives you a confidence boost. Go through the practice tests until you feel comfortable, and then you can go into the test knowing that you're ready for it.

Test Tips

On test day, you should be confident, knowing that you've prepared well and are ready to answer the questions. But aside from preparation, there are several test day strategies you can employ to maximize your performance.

First, as stated before, get a good night's sleep the night before the test (and for several nights before that, if possible). Go into the test with a fresh, alert mind rather than staying up late to study.

Try not to change too much about your normal routine on the day of the test. It's important to eat a nutritious breakfast, but if you normally don't eat breakfast at all, consider eating just a protein bar. If you're a coffee drinker, go ahead and have your normal coffee. Just make sure you time it so that the caffeine doesn't wear off right in the middle of your test. Avoid sugary beverages, and drink enough water to stay hydrated but not so much that you need a restroom break 10 minutes into the test. If your test isn't first thing in the morning, consider going for a walk or doing a light workout before the test to get your blood flowing.

Allow yourself enough time to get ready, and leave for the test with plenty of time to spare so you won't have the anxiety of scrambling to arrive in time. Another reason to be early is to select a good seat. It's helpful to sit away from doors and windows, which can be distracting. Find a good seat, get out your supplies, and settle your mind before the test begins.

When the test begins, start by going over the instructions carefully, even if you already know what to expect. Make sure you avoid any careless mistakes by following the directions.

Then begin working through the questions, pacing yourself as you've practiced. If you're not sure on an answer, don't spend too much time on it, and don't let it shake your confidence. Either skip it and come back later, or eliminate as many wrong answers as possible and guess among the remaining ones. Don't dwell on these questions as you continue—put them out of your mind and focus on what lies ahead.

Be sure to read all of the answer choices, even if you're sure the first one is the right answer. Sometimes you'll find a better one if you keep reading. But don't second-guess yourself if you do immediately know the answer. Your gut instinct is usually right. Don't let test anxiety rob you of the information you know.

If you have time at the end of the test (and if the test format allows), go back and review your answers. Be cautious about changing any, since your first instinct tends to be correct, but make sure you didn't misread any of the questions or accidentally mark the wrong answer choice. Look over any you skipped and make an educated guess.

At the end, leave the test feeling confident. You've done your best, so don't waste time worrying about your performance or wishing you could change anything. Instead, celebrate the successful completion of this test. And finally, use this test to learn how to deal with anxiety even better next time.

> **Review Video: Test Anxiety**
> Visit mometrix.com/academy and enter code: 100340

Important Qualification

Not all anxiety is created equal. If your test anxiety is causing major issues in your life beyond the classroom or testing center, or if you are experiencing troubling physical symptoms related to your anxiety, it may be a sign of a serious physiological or psychological condition. If this sounds like your situation, we strongly encourage you to seek professional help.

Online Resources

Due to our efforts to try to keep this book to a manageable length, we've created a link that will give you access to all of your online resources:

mometrix.com/resources719/ardmssonoprin

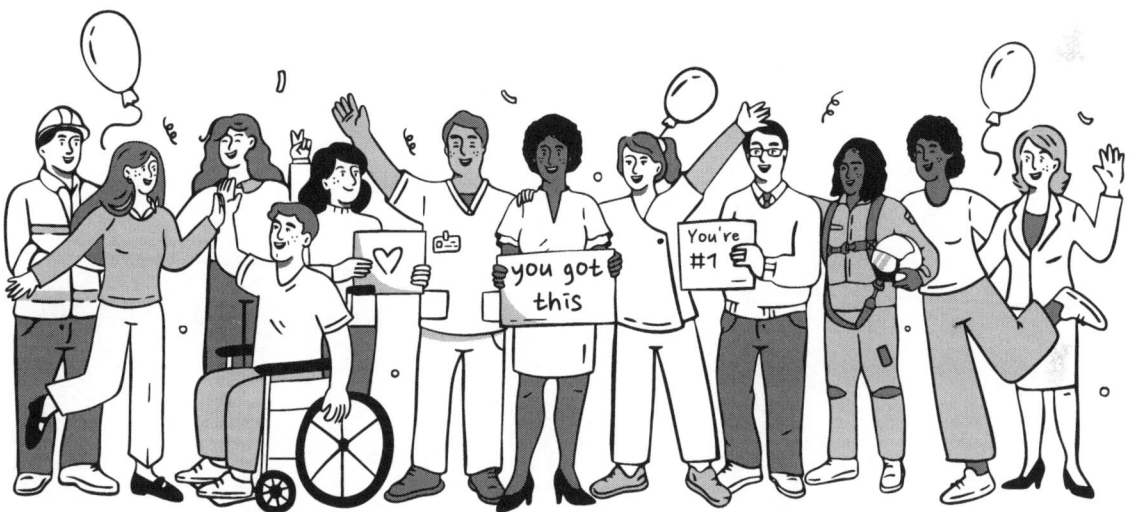